Rachael Holme was born a̶n̶ originally trained in London as a beautician and remedial therapist, but left that profession to set up a natural food shop, restaurant and bakery with her husband, Peter. Her enthusiasm for cooking with wholefoods and her experience gained as a professional cook in their restaurant led her to write natural food cookery books, and so far she has published *Better Breakfasts*; *Baking Better Breads*; *Cakes, Scones and Biscuits*; and *Natural Spices*. When her own children were conceived and born she combined her practical knowledge of good nutrition and healthy eating with her experience of pregnancy and birth, and has since set out to make others more aware of the important connections between good pre-conception care and diet and the birth of healthy babies. She is now a freelance writer and has contributed articles to various magazines. She has also broadcast on radio. She lives in Cambridgeshire with her husband and three children.

Miriam Polunin

RACHAEL HOLME

Pregnancy and Diet

PENGUIN BOOKS

Penguin Books Ltd, Harmondsworth, Middlesex, England
Viking Penguin Inc., 40 West 23rd Street, New York, New York 10010, U.S.A.
Penguin Books Australia Ltd, Ringwood, Victoria, Australia
Penguin Books Canada Ltd, 2801 John Street, Markham, Ontario, Canada L3R 1B4
Penguin Books (N.Z.) Ltd, 182–190 Wairau Road, Auckland 10, New Zealand

First published 1985

Printed and bound in Great Britain by
Cox & Wyman Ltd, Reading
Filmset in Trump (Linotron 202) by
Rowland Phototypesetting Ltd,
Bury St Edmunds, Suffolk

This book is dedicated to
our third baby,
Thomas Edward,
conceived and born during the writing of it,
who played a more prominent part in the research for this work
than he will ever know.

It is also dedicated to my husband Peter
and our two older children Daniel and Rosie,
for their enduring support and inspiring qualities.

Contents

Contents

List of Text Figures

Gaining Weight in Pregnancy

A weighty problem?

The very nature of the state of pregnancy makes a woman gain weight during the forty weeks she is carrying her child. There are many women who start pregnancy at around the desirable weight for their height, but some are too heavy before conceiving and others are too thin from the start. These two extremes are both considered unhealthy environments for a growing foetus. A grossly overweight pregnant woman runs many extra health risks (see p. 17, 'How excess weight in pregnancy could affect you'), while a seriously underweight mother-to-be is more likely to give birth to an underweight baby, and small babies can suffer serious complications after they are born. It must be stressed that women who are only a few pounds over or under their desirable weight have no need to worry. It is only if you are an extreme case that you need special attention, and your doctor will diagnose this for himself. If you are concerned that you may be bordering on either of these two extreme categories, talk to your doctor as soon as possible and ask his advice. He will either reassure you, or give you some advice about your condition and possibly refer you to a specialist. Even if you do fall into one of these two categories this does not necessarily mean that you will experience more difficulties during your pregnancy than a woman whose weight is normal, but it does mean that your progress may need to be monitored closely to minimize any possible risks. To find out what your desirable weight for your height and frame size should be, turn to p. 13.

It you are not yet pregnant but want to start a baby soon, and are concerned that you may be over or underweight, talk to your doctor now. If your doctor thinks it is wise for you to gain or lose some weight, you can do so under his expert supervision before conceiving. If you need to lose weight, which is by far the most common case, you will find that most doctors are willing to give you helpful dietary advice and will usually also offer calorie charts and back-up literature about slimming. This could be just the incentive you need to succeed, even if you have unsuccessfully tried to lose weight before. Starting your pregnancy at the correct weight will be beneficial to both you and your baby, and will diminish the possibility of any serious complications during pregnancy and afterwards.

If you are already pregnant and are too thin, you may find that pregnancy is just the right treatment you need to build you up. You may find that because you are pregnant your appetite will improve, so that you will be eating enough to increase your own weight as well as providing the extra nourishment for your growing baby. If this is the case with you, make sure you feed your appetite with the right ingredients nutritionally (see Chapters 2 and 4).

If, on the other hand, you are already overweight and pregnant too, you may be horrified to find that this maternal condition you find yourself in makes you fatter than ever, and possibly more quickly than is usually thought reasonable. If the thought of the weeks and months ahead and of your ever-increasing bulk frightens you, don't be too miserable at this stage. Although it is not advisable to try to lose weight while pregnant (except on special advice from your doctor), you can minimize the dangers and damage of extra poundage by eating carefully from now on, to make sure that you avoid putting on any *more* than the normally accepted 26–30 lb during the nine months you are carrying your child. Make sure the food you do eat is nutritionally good. Don't eat high calorie foods which are low in nutritional value. See Chapter 4 for advice on which foods fill the bill. Just because you are a bit plump to start with, that is not an excuse to chomp away on chocolates and cakes because you think it won't make much difference. It will. Don't make excuses for over-eating, but find ways to limit your weight gain to the acceptable average, or slightly below. This book will help you. Start to plan ahead now for after the baby's birth, when you will want very much to be slim again. Think positively and you will succeed.

A growing concern

Most women are concerned in some respect about their weight when they find themselves pregnant for the first time. Usually this takes the form of worrying that they will turn into fat, flabby and obese mothers who will never be able to return to their former slenderness. While this is generally an unreasonable fear, take care – some do. Make sure you are not one of them by planning your diet sensibly now. It is not surprising that so many women worry about extra weight that pregnancy brings when we consider the rate at which a mother-to-be piles on the pounds. At first the weight gain doesn't seem too bad, not more than 2 lb per month for the first five months (10 lb maximum altogether). This first increase in weight need not make very much difference to your appearance, although some women find that they tend to 'blow up' with very swollen breasts and tummy at this stage. Although this may be very noticeable to you, most other people won't be aware of it, and most pregnancies can easily be disguised for about four months if you are shy about your condition. I think this is a shame, because if you are pregnant it's nice to show it. However, there are many women who don't agree, so it is reassuring to know that you can choose to flaunt your condition or not to start with, just as the fancy takes you when the time comes. Whatever you decide, try to keep your weight gain for the first five months at around 10 lb by eating thoughtfully, with good nutrition in mind, and then you will be able to congratulate yourself and look forward to the following months with confidence.

Although you have been recommended to keep between certain weight limits during your pregnancy (guidelines only), it is difficult for several reasons to be more specific about the *rate* of extra poundage you should expect. Firstly, pregnancy is gauged by weeks, forty altogether. However, forty weeks do not conveniently divide into nine equal parts, or nine months, so the third and sixth months are regarded as containing six weeks each. This may seem awkward at first, but it does make sense if you follow it through because it means that the extra four weeks which do not fit into the nine months are absorbed into the first two-thirds of pregnancy, thus allowing the last third (which is the most important as far as confirming your expected date of confinement is concerned) to be accurately counted in weeks (see Fig. 1).

Secondly, because it is unusual to know the exact date of conception, the expected date of delivery is calculated from the first day of your last period. This can be muddling, as it means including the two weeks or so after the beginning of your period when you were not actually pregnant, although this is allowed for in the calculation. The most likely time for conception is midway between two menstrual periods, but in fact the date of conception can vary enormously, especially if you are one of those women whose menstrual periods are not regular 28-day cycles. Use Fig. 2 to help you work out as accurately as possible your expected date of delivery, based on the first day of your last period. If you haven't kept a record of the dates of your period it will be even more difficult to calculate your expected date of delivery, but your doctor will be able to make a fairly accurate guess by noting monthly the change in size of the uterus. In order to be really accurate an ultrasound scan can be taken at about 16 weeks, and this may be advised for you if you are unsure of your dates.

Lastly, women gain weight in pregnancy at different rates, but most still manage to even out at a total gain of around 2 stone. While most women gain more weight at the end of pregnancy, there are a few who gain more at the beginning and less towards the end. So if you don't fit exactly into the stereotype mother-to-be mould, don't worry – we are all

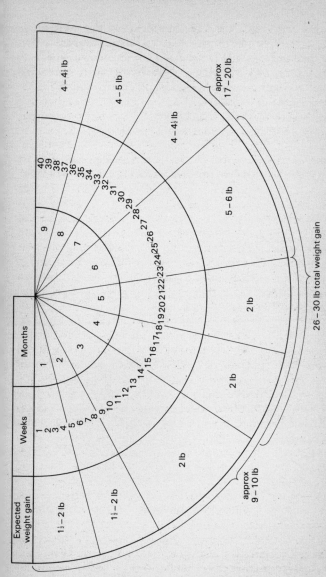

Expected weight gain	Weeks	Months
1½ – 2 lb	1 2 3 4	1
1½ – 2 lb	5 6 7 8 9 10	2 3
2 lb	11 12 13 14	4 5 6
2 lb	15 16 17 18 19 20 21 22 23 24 25 26 27 28	7 8 9
2 lb		
4 – 4½ lb	29 30 31 32 33 34 35 36 37 38 39 40	
4 – 5 lb		
4 – 4½ lb		
5 – 6 lb		

approx 9 – 10 lb

26 – 30 lb total weight gain

approx 17 – 20 lb

Fig. 1. How the weeks of pregnancy are divided into months, and the average weight gain by the mother for each month.

individuals, with different lifestyles, and the results that these variations bring are bound to differ slightly. No two women start off with the same figure, and the visual effects of pregnancy are bound to be different too. Fig. 3 gives you a general idea of how you can expect the pounds to show during the nine months.

Weighing the balance

So what about all this extra weight you are going to be carrying? Exactly how much should you gain? It is obvious

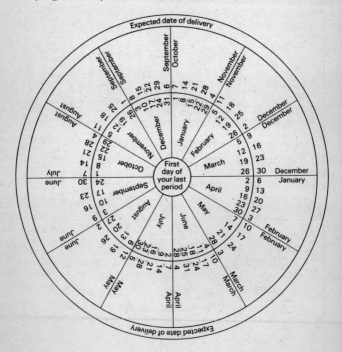

Fig. 2. *Expected date of delivery in relation to the first day of your last period. Dates on the inside circle represent the first day of your last period, dates on the outside circle represent corresponding expected dates of delivery.*

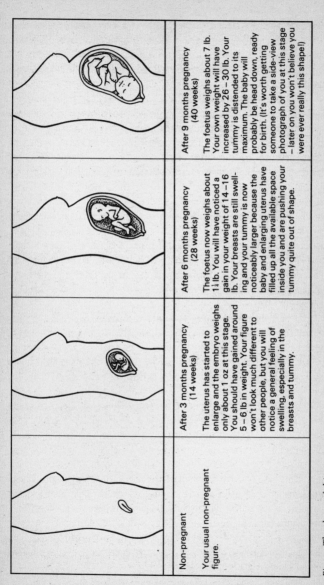

Non-pregnant	After 3 months pregnancy (14 weeks)	After 6 months pregnancy (28 weeks)	After 9 months pregnancy (40 weeks)
Your usual non-pregnant figure.	The uterus has started to enlarge and the embryo weighs only about 1 oz at this stage. You should have gained around 5 – 6 lb in weight. Your figure won't look much different to other people, but you will notice a general feeling of swelling, especially in the breasts and tummy.	The foetus now weighs about 1½ lb. You will have noticed a gain in your weight of 14 –16 lb. Your breasts are still swelling and your tummy is now noticeably larger because the baby and enlarging uterus have filled up all the available space inside you and are pushing your tummy quite out of shape.	The foetus weighs about 7 lb. Your own weight will have increased by 26 – 30 lb. Your tummy is distended to its maximum. The baby will probably be head down, ready for birth. (It's worth getting someone to take a side-view photograph of you at this stage – later on you won't believe you were ever really this shape!)

Fig. 3. *The shape of things to come.*

that a pregnant woman's weight is going to increase, but the vital questions to ask are precisely how much, and why? There are several factors involved in calculating the total amount, so let's start at the beginning with the development of the baby itself.

Most people know that the average weight of a new-born baby is around 7 lb, but there can be enormous variations in this figure. I know of one mother who delivered a 12-lb baby, but I also know of another whose premature twins weighed only around 2 lb at birth. All three babies grew up to be healthy, intelligent children, emphasizing the fact that it is the maturity of the foetus that counts, not its size. It is interesting to note that just as the mother's weight increase occurs in leaps and bounds over the nine months of pregnancy, so does her baby's. A foetus in the womb doesn't gain weight in conveniently equal amounts each month – it has various different spurts of growth according to whether it is growing and developing organs, as in early pregnancy, or maturing and laying down layers of fat beneath its skin, as happens later.

In a normal pregnancy, the sperm joins up with the egg to form the embryo somewhere along the fallopian tube. The fertilized egg, which at this stage is still so small that it cannot be seen with the naked eye, spends the next four days or so making its way down the fallopian tube to the uterus. Here it embeds itself into the wall of the uterus and starts to grow. It is recognizable as a tiny, living being by the time it is about six weeks old, although it is still so small that you can't feel it inside you. It is still only about half an inch long, and at this stage the placenta is usually bigger than the embryo itself. Two weeks later the embryo is twice as long (an inch). At twelve weeks the foetus will weigh around half an ounce, and all the major organs in its body will have formed. At sixteen weeks it will have increased its weight to around 4 oz. By the time twenty weeks have passed it will have nearly trebled its weight yet again, to around 12 oz. The foetus continues to grow at a startling rate now, tipping the scales at 1½ lb after twenty-four weeks. Four weeks later it will be over 2 lb in weight. At thirty-two weeks it will weigh around 3½–4 lb, at least half its final birthweight. The next four weeks sees a very large increase as it starts to lay down fat under its skin, and it now reaches around 5 or 6 lb. By the end of pregnancy, at forty weeks, it has reached its final birthweight of around 7–7½ lbs. Boys are often a few ounces heavier at birth than girls.

So if the baby itself accounts for only about a quarter of the weight that the mother gains, what makes up the other three-quarters of the total weight? The baby is surrounded in the womb by the amniotic fluid or 'waters', which at full term can amount to 1½–2 pints. This fluid and the placenta, which is the baby's lifeline through which it receives all the nourishment it needs for its successful growth in the womb, probably account for another 3 lb or so.

The walls of the uterus must become strong enough to contain the growing baby, the amniotic fluid and the placenta for the required length of time. The uterine walls therefore expand and thicken greatly to provide a nourishing environment for the growth of the baby – before pregnancy the uterus is about 3 inches long and is positioned between the bladder and the rectum, but after forty weeks of pregnancy the top of the uterus has expanded and lifted up into the abdominal cavity, and the whole uterus is nearer 12 inches long. At the same time the breasts enlarge and swell and start to prepare for producing milk. At first, when you are only just pregnant, your breasts will feel tender and possibly tingle, being extra sensitive to touch. As pregnancy progresses they will start to swell and increase in size, as the ducts and alveoli (the minute sacs which make up the secreting part of the mammary gland) grow and enlarge to make themselves ready for lactation. By the end of pregnancy a normally small bust, say 32 inches, could increase up to 36 inches. This extra weight, combined with that of the enlarged uterus, can account for another 2–3 lb.

The next factor to take into consideration is that fat is

much more easily laid down in the body during pregnancy. In the normal course of events, any excess carbohydrate eaten is turned into fat and laid down in the tissues of the body. A pregnant woman, however, secretes certain hormones which have the effect of *increasing* the amount of fat that is laid down. This is almost certainly nature's way of making sure that there will be a sufficient store of fat in the mother's body to be drawn on for feeding the baby in the early weeks of life. In prehistoric times this would have been vital, allowing the mother to have a chance to recover from the birth for a few days or so before needing to forage for food again. It is a left-over mechanism of nature, a trick of evolution to help ensure the success of the species. Mothers who choose to breastfeed almost always find that, even though they may be eating large amounts of food, this extra weight disappears fairly quickly after the birth simply because the store of fat that was laid down is being used in the way it was intended – to feed the baby. Mothers who choose to bottle-feed their babies very often find it much harder to shift excess weight once the baby is born, because the store of fat is not being used.

Extra water is also retained in the mother's body throughout pregnancy, most noticeably in the second half, between twenty and forty weeks. The actual increase in the amount of water in the body at full term surprises many women – it can be as much as 6 or 7 pints. This amount of extra liquid can account for another 8 or 9 lb in weight. The extra fat and the extra liquid are both laid down because of increased hormone levels.

Finally, because the mother's blood system is having to perform all the tasks necessary for the continued life and growth of the baby, such as supplying it with oxygen and nutrients and carrying away its waste products, as well as coping with her own needs, the volume of blood in the mother's body increases. This extra blood can account for another 2–3 lb in weight.

The combination of all these factors results in an accepted weight gain in pregnancy of between 26 and 30 lb in total (see

Fig. 4). You can see that most of the extra weight is due to the formation of the various support systems inside your body which keep your baby alive and well, with only a small amount being due to extra fat. So it is obvious that in order to build the best and healthiest placenta, umbilical cord and other supporting components of pregnancy, so that the baby you produce is as healthy as possible and gets the best start in life you can physically give him, it is very important to think carefully about your diet and eat the right foods to do the job

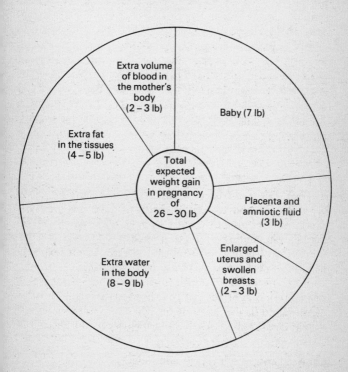

Fig. 4. Contributing factors affecting the total expected weight gain in pregnancy.

FIG. 5. *Expected weight gain at two stages of pregnancy, in relation to height.*

Height (without shoes)			Normal non-pregnant weight			Expected maximum weight after 20 weeks pregnancy (4½ months)			Expected maximum weight at 40 weeks pregnancy (9 months)		
ft	ins	m	st	lb	kg	st	lb	kg	st	lb	kg
4	11	1.50	7	12	50.0	8	8	54.5	10	0	63.5
5	0	1.52	8	1	51.3	8	11	55.8	10	3	65.0
5	1	1.55	8	4	52.5	9	0	57.0	10	6	66.2
5	2	1.57	8	7	54.0	9	3	58.5	10	9	67.5
5	3	1.60	8	10	55.5	9	6	60.0	10	12	69.0
5	4	1.63	9	0	57.0	9	10	61.5	11	2	70.8
5	5	1.65	9	4	59.0	10	0	63.5	11	6	72.5
5	6	1.68	9	9	61.7	10	5	65.8	11	11	75.0
5	7	1.70	9	13	63.0	10	9	67.5	12	1	76.5
5	8	1.73	10	3	65.0	10	13	69.5	12	5	78.5
5	9	1.75	10	7	66.5	11	3	71.2	12	9	80.0
5	10	1.78	10	11	68.5	11	7	73.0	12	13	81.5
5	11	1.80	11	1	70.5	11	11	75.0	13	3	84.0
6	0	1.83	11	5	72.0	12	1	76.5	13	7	85.7

properly. Good nutrition is important in order to produce a healthy baby and to ensure that you have the necessary energy and stamina to see you through the delivery and the first few demanding weeks after birth.

Fig. 5 will help you visualize the rate of your expected weight gain more easily. The weights given are for a woman with a medium frame, and are only approximate. If you have a small frame, subtract up to 9 lb from each weight measurement. If you have a large frame, add on up to 12 lb for each weight measurement. Do be honest with yourself about this.

Knowing how much you should weigh

It is useful to know whether you are starting your pregnancy weighing the correct or 'desirable' amount. If you are already pregnant and know your weight before conceiving, you can still judge whether you started pregnancy within the ideal weight boundaries set down in Fig. 6. (Remember, though, that the tables are only a guide – don't worry if your weight before conceiving is not *exactly* the same as that set out in the table, as long as it is fairly close.) Most of us, if we are honest with ourselves, know whether we are a bit on the large side, but it is useful to be able to check on a chart to confirm our beliefs. Don't forget to measure your height without shoes, and weigh yourself without clothes, otherwise the result will not be accurate.

Fig. 6 gives approximate desirable weights for women according to height and frame. If you are not sure which frame size you belong to, consider yourself to be medium.

FIG. 6. *Approximate desirable weights for women before conceiving, in relation to height and frame size. (Remember that these 'desirable' weights are only approximate, and if you weigh a few pounds over or under you need not be concerned. Measure your height without shoes and weigh yourself without clothes.)*

Height			Small frame			Medium frame			Large frame		
ft	ins	m	st	lb	kg	st	lb	kg	st	lb	kg
4	11	1.50	7	3	46.0	7	12	50.0	8	10	55.5
5	0	1.52	7	6	47.0	8	1	51.3	8	13	56.5
5	1	1.55	7	9	48.5	8	4	52.5	9	2	58.0
5	2	1.57	7	12	50.0	8	7	54.0	9	5	59.5
5	3	1.60	8	1	51.3	8	10	55.5	9	8	61.0
5	4	1.63	8	5	53.0	9	0	57.0	9	12	62.5
5	5	1.65	8	9	54.8	9	4	59.0	10	2	64.5
5	6	1.68	9	0	57.0	9	9	61.7	10	7	66.5
5	7	1.70	9	4	59.0	9	13	63.0	10	11	68.5
5	8	1.73	9	8	61.0	10	3	65.0	11	1	70.5
5	9	1.75	9	12	62.5	10	7	66.5	11	5	72.0
5	10	1.78	10	2	64.5	10	11	68.5	11	9	74.0
5	11	1.80	10	6	66.2	11	1	70.5	11	13	75.8
6	0	1.83	10	10	68.0	11	5	72.0	12	3	77.5

Don't worry too much if you are a couple of pounds over the desirable weight shown – people are built differently, and slight variations in weight for women of the same height are normal. If, however, you find that you are more than 10 lb over the desirable weight before conceiving, you should consider yourself to be a bit too heavy. (Similarly, if you find that you are more than 10 lb lighter than your desirable weight before conceiving, you should consider yourself to be quite thin enough.) This kind of variation in weight is fairly common and not dangerous, but if you are 10 lb overweight it may be an indication that you are prone to holding on to any excess calories you eat. If you are in this category it is a good idea to be more aware of your diet, and especially to avoid sugary or fatty foods while you are pregnant, so that your weight will not increase too much beyond the accepted level. This does not mean that you need to 'go on a diet' in the conventional sense, it merely means that it would be wise for you to make sure that all the food you do consume is the right sort of body-building, energy-giving, healthy food that you need. It is not so much a question of cutting down on your food (unless you are already eating too much in the first place), but rather a matter of exchanging the less nutritious parts of your diet (too much sugar, too much fat, white flour products) for more nourishing alternatives – a much smaller amount of sugary things, or fruit or honey instead, a more moderate portion of fat (we all need a little in our diet), and wholewheat products which contain more fibre. In this way you will be starting to make your diet much healthier. You will soon find, too, that it is more difficult to over-eat with these sorts of foods – it is difficult to eat too much fresh fruit, whereas it is terribly easy to eat too much cake. Wholewheat, fibre-full foods are more filling than their white alternatives, so you will tend to eat less of them. Ways in which you can moderate your diet to make it healthier and more suitable for pregnancy are enlarged on in Chapter 4.

It is only women who are dangerously overweight and pregnant who need special care and treatment from their doctors. Real obesity is not all that common; you would need to be enormously heavier than your recommended weight to come into that category. But plumpness is very much more common, and if you tend towards being plump it is just as well to be aware of the situation so that you can watch your weight gain carefully while you are pregnant.

Overweight and overwhelmed?

At this point you may well exclaim that this is all very well provided you are near the correct, desirable weight to begin with. If you are, well and good, you will be able to follow the chapters on nutrition and good diet in pregnancy without concerning yourself too much about excess weight. All you will have to do is make sure that you don't put on *more* weight than is desirable. (If you find you are gaining weight too quickly, you can follow some of the ideas for moderating your diet calorie-wise without forgoing good nutrition (pp. 21–3), or read Chapter 4 for ideas to help you to make your diet more balanced.)

But what happens if you are already far heavier than your desirable weight and want a baby? Or if you are already pregnant and overweight, and desperately concerned that the next nine months will see an even bigger increase in your weight which you fear you may never be able to lose again afterwards? Well, don't panic, because help is at hand. If you come into either of these two categories, read on, stop worrying, and do something positive about it now.

First those of you who are not yet pregnant: if you are overweight and considering conceiving a baby soon, please turn to Chapters 3 and 4, which are about preconception care and diet, and read them very carefully *before you conceive*. If you are overweight it is a good idea to try to lose some of the excess before you become pregnant at all. Try to ensure that you don't just read these two chapters, but that you act on them too, for the benefit of yourself and your new baby.

If, however, you are overweight and already pregnant, start thinking about your diet in a new way (read Chapter 4 and apply it to your pregnancy now). Think about what you are eating, and stay away from over-rich, fatty or sugary foods in an effort to keep your expected weight gain normal. Although it must be emphasized that a woman should never actively try to *lose* weight while pregnant (except on the direct advice of her doctor), there are lots of helpful, positive, useful things you can do to minimize the danger of becoming fatter than ever while you are carrying your baby. If you scan through any slimming magazine, you will soon discover the uncomfortable fact that the majority of women who are trying to shift excess fat complain that pregnancy had an awful lot to do with their present weighty condition. Most of them blame pregnancy for at least part if not all of their weight problem. This is not because pregnancy itself is 'fattening', but because they did not know how to adapt to their new condition, were not told in advance of the care they should take with their diet while pregnant, and did not know what level of weight increase in pregnancy was acceptable. How much better it would have been for those women if they had not accumulated all that extra fat during their pregnancies in the first place. So, if you are overweight and pregnant too, the first thing you can do to help yourself is to make sure that throughout your pregnancy you do not put on any *more* weight than the generally accepted increase. Then, when your baby is born, you will be able to think about reducing your weight further without having very much excess fat left over from pregnancy to make things even more difficult for you.

Food can be fun

Don't regard the task of watching what you eat during pregnancy as being boring or difficult, because really it is neither of these. Food can be fun; making sure you are eating well for the sake of yourself and your baby can be satisfying and rewarding, if only because you will know that you are doing your very best to ensure that your baby has the best possible environmental conditions in which to grow and thrive inside you until birth. You will also know that you are taking care of yourself at the same time, and can look forward to the time after the baby's birth knowing that weight-wise and figure-wise you will be no worse off than before you conceived. If you tend to worry about your figure anyway this should be very helpful to you, so stop worrying and start taking care of your diet from now on. Monitor your diet carefully with good nutrition in mind. You can ensure that, while your diet contains adequate calories for your condition, you are eating healthy, nutritious food which will provide you with all the necessary protein, fibre, vitamins and minerals for you and your baby, and not sugary, refined, junk foods that will not help you, your baby, or your future figure.

How excess weight in pregnancy could affect you

It is useful to know about some of the problems that excess weight in pregnancy can bring, if only to give you extra incentive to stay within the accepted weight levels. Gross obesity coupled with pregnancy is a recipe for disaster as far as health is concerned. Fortunately, although many of us are a bit overweight, really gross obesity is a fairly rare occurrence. Indeed, there is some evidence to suggest that obese women are in such a poor state of health that they are unlikely to conceive at all, which is just as well, since an obese woman's body is under such stress due to her excess bulk that it is very unlikely it would be able to cope properly with the added strains and stresses and demands made by a growing baby. It has also been said that obese mothers often have a longer labour than normal, and have trouble breast-feeding.

Certain medical conditions which may crop up in pregnancy can be made very much worse if you are seriously overweight as well. One such condition is oedema (swelling of the hands, face and ankles). Another is high blood pressure. Varicose veins can also be made very much worse – these are at best unsightly and can cause uncomfortable aches in the legs. Toxaemia (a particularly lethal combination of high blood pressure, general swelling in the body and the occurrence of protein in the urine, which in its severest form can cause fits or convulsions in the mother and the likely death of the baby) is most certainly linked with excess weight, so it really is worth trying to keep your weight gain in pregnancy within safe limits.

Helping yourself

If, after having looked at the height/weight chart on p. 13, you decide that you were perhaps a bit on the heavy side before conceiving, here are a few ideas to help you stay within the recommended weight gain levels for pregnancy of 26–30 lb in all. These ideas are aimed at generally making your diet more nutritious, healthy and balanced, while at the same time avoiding 'empty' calories, or those foods which provide lots of calories but little nutritional value. The aim is not to cut down on calories (unless you are really eating more than you need anyway), but rather to ensure that the food you do consume is the best, healthiest, most nutritious and most beneficial sort.

Three old wives' tales to ignore

There are many superstitions, mistaken beliefs and old wives' tales surrounding all aspects of pregnancy and delivery. While there may be a grain of truth in one or two of them, I think it best in general to ignore what most often turns out to be unsubstantiated rumour. Three old wives' tales in particular, concerning diet in pregnancy, should definitely be ignored.

1. Don't believe that you need to eat for two while you are pregnant. While it is true that you will need a little extra of most things in your diet, it must be emphasized that it will only be a *little* more, and it certainly won't amount to double your normal intake of food.
2. Don't eat away contentedly, thinking to yourself that any

extra weight you may put on while pregnant will somehow all miraculously drop off again by itself after the baby is born. *It won't.* You would be fooling yourself if you took comfort in this idea. Too many calories *always* equals too much fat laid down in the body. This holds good before pregnancy, during pregnancy and after pregnancy. Having a baby doesn't magically alter your metabolism so that your body automatically uses up everything you eat.

3. If you have been in the habit of over-eating before pregnancy and are therefore rather overweight when your pregnancy begins, don't allow yourself to continue over-eating while carrying your baby just because you think 'I am too fat anyway so it won't make much difference.' This is just an excuse, though it is often used. If you were already a bit too heavy before conceiving, that is *all the more reason* to avoid compounding the problem now.

Thinking about the calories you eat

There are lots of people who never give a second thought to what they are eating and how their food is converted into energy. Some people, the lucky ones, don't need to because their appetite corresponds exactly to their calorific needs. This is the ideal situation, the slimmer's dream, when your hunger is adequately satisfied by eating just the right amount of food to give you the energy you need each day. Under these circumstances the energy you are taking in is exactly equalled by the energy you are giving out, with the happy result that you neither gain nor lose any weight. However, one of the common side effects of pregnancy is that your appetite may increase, sometimes beyond your dietary needs, and if you find this noticeably happening to you, it may be very interesting to find out just how much more you are eating.

First of all, get into the habit of roughly counting the calories you consume each day. Write down everything you eat in a notebook, at the time you eat it (it's surprising how easily you can 'forget' about a mid-morning snack), and then work out the calorific value, using the chart on p. 200 of this book. Then add up the grand total at the end of the day. You may be surprised to find that you are eating more than you need. If the total is somewhere around 2,000 calories per day, you are obviously on the right track. But if your daily total is more than 2,400 calories, you should make an effort to curb your appetite or you may find that your weight will increase too fast. It should not be difficult to stay below this level – it really is quite a generous amount of food each day, as any slimmer will tell you.

FIG. 7. *Approximate daily calorie requirements for women of childbearing age.*

Slimmer on a weight reducing diet	1000–1500
Non-pregnant woman, and pregnant woman during the first 3 months of pregnancy	1700–2100
Pregnant woman during the last six months of pregnancy	2000–2400
Breastfeeding woman	up to 2700

Note: A woman with a very inactive lifestyle will have a calorie requirement at the lower level given, whereas a physically active woman will need the higher levels. It will be noticed that calorie requirements during the first three months of pregnancy do not differ very much from normal, whereas approximately 300 extra calories per day are required during the last six months of pregnancy.

It is also useful to be able to work out more accurately just what your calorie requirement is likely to be. You know that, roughly speaking, it should not be less than 1,700 or more than 2,400 calories each day while you are pregnant. To find out your own personal calorific requirement between these two figures, you must take into consideration the type of lifestyle you have and your daily activities. Be honest about just how active you are. Pregnancy often has the effect of making you very sleepy and inactive to begin with. If you find yourself taking long naps in the afternoon and generally taking things easy, your calorie requirement is likely to be nearer the lower level. If, however, you already have a demanding toddler to care for, or other children at school to organize, or a part-time or full-time job, your calorific requirement may be nearer the upper limit.

Don't consider yourself to be 'on a diet'. You are merely taking stock of the situation and reviewing your eating habits with a view to improving the quality of your diet for your health's sake.

The food itself

What makes up a healthy diet and constitutes good nutrition is discussed at greater length in Chapters 2 and 4. Here are a few basic ideas to set you on your way in the meantime. Don't try to adjust everything in your diet simultaneously or you will find it too strange and difficult. Instead, make a point of taking things one step at a time. After you have become used to one dietary change, think about adding the next one to your repertoire. Don't keep all this to yourself either – these are general, health-conscious food tips for everyone, and are of just as much benefit to husbands and children as they are to expectant mothers. Experimenting with your diet and trying out new ideas is much more fun and less boring if you have other people to discuss it with. If you encourage everyone in the family to join in it will also be easier to control in the kitchen – you will not need to prepare any special meals for yourself, and you can all be healthier together. Make these changes permanent for all the family.

Making a start

Changing your diet for the better is easy, and what's more, it can be fun and interesting too. People are always asking me the best way to begin making a change, and how to keep their new diet varied enough to keep all the family happy. Some people's diets are so boring it's unbelievable. Some families have the same old fare on the table day after day. Many people have trouble thinking up enough imaginative meals and therefore find food boring. And it *is* boring, unhealthy and unadventurous to serve up the same meals time and time again. If you follow the plan of campaign in this book to outlaw processed and refined foods from your kitchen this problem will disappear, because there is a huge range of healthy, nutritious, natural foods to choose from, available all year round. Follow these simple rules and make a start slowly. Try out the ideas one by one. Further help about changing your diet is given in Chapter 4. Soon you will find that you won't want to return to your boring old culinary routine, as the food you eat will *taste* so much better anyway.

Ten basic tips for a healthier diet

1. Variety is the spice of life, and one of the secrets of a really healthy diet. Make sure you eat foods from as wide a range of products as possible, so that you get a good balance of proteins, carbohydrates, fats, vitamins and minerals. Don't be afraid to try new foods. Experiment with tastes and textures. If you find one particular food you particularly like, trying cooking it in lots of different ways.

2. Try to cut down on all obviously refined, processed foods and replace them wherever you can with fresh alternatives. First of all eliminate all ready-made puddings, cake mixes and commercial confectionery.

3. Make a point of checking the ingredients list on any ready-made food product you do buy. If sugar or fat comes near the top of the list, or if it contains a wide variety of colourings, artificial flavourings and preservatives, discard it and use a fresh alternative.

4. Cut down on processed meats of all kinds and replace them with fresh cuts of meat and offal. Many processed meat products contain chemicals such as polysulphates, which allow the meat to retain more water and thereby increase the manufacturer's profits. Similarly, cut down on processed fish products and use fresh or frozen whole fish instead.

5. Eat a good variety of fresh fruit and fresh vegetables, including green vegetables, each day. Try to eat some of your

vegetables raw in salads, as this way they retain many more of their valuable nutrients.

6. Give up white, refined flour products and substitute wholewheat products which contain more fibre. Wholewheat flour and wholewheat bread are now available everywhere, and do not cost much more than the white variety. Wholewheat pasta, especially brown spaghetti and macaroni, are also becoming much more widely available, even in supermarkets. Brown rice is much better for you than white rice, and tastes better too – it has a crunchy, nutty flavour.

7. Try to cut down as much as you can, or cut out altogether, any sugary products such as cakes, biscuits, sweets and chocolates. Replace them with fresh fruit, dried fruits (which are very sweet), and honey-based recipes.

8. Use fresh dairy products wherever possible. Fresh milk, live yogurt, and low and medium fat cheeses are fine. Go easy on cream, butter and full fat cheeses. Don't use processed, sliced cheeses or sugar-filled commercial yogurts.

9. Include dried pulses, beans and lentils in your diet. They are a cheap source of protein, and contain plenty of fibre to help bulk out your diet and fill you up. Beans can be used to make more expensive fresh cuts of meat go further.

10. Cut down on fried, fatty foods. Instead of frying an egg, poach it or boil it. Instead of making chips, try a baked potato. Meat and fish can be grilled instead of fried, and they retain a better flavour this way too.

You need not try putting all these ideas into practice in the order they are written here. First choose the one you think you are most likely to succeed with, then gradually add the others one by one.

Pregnant and plump too?

For those of you who are pregnant and know full well that you were a bit on the heavy side before conceiving, here are a few more words of encouragement. Your pregnancy need not add to your existing weight problem if you follow the advice here. As you start to attend your antenatal clinic you will probably find that there are many other women just like you. It seems in particular that women carrying their second baby are quite likely to start off too heavy, probably because they never managed to lose the extra weight they may have gained during their first pregnancy. Although this doesn't necessarily happen to everybody, I know for sure that it is quite a common occurrence just by looking around and talking to other mothers. It is all too easy, once your first baby is born, to take the attitude that because you will probably be wanting another one shortly (the majority of couples aim for at least two children), you might as well forget about your figure until you've finished reproducing altogether. This of course is untrue and misleading, but it is one area where husbands or partners can be very helpful indeed – by reminding you (gently, of course) that it is worth struggling a bit to get your figure back between babies, and to return to your desirable weight so that you will begin your next pregnancy with confidence, weight-wise.

If you are plump and pregnant too, I think one of the best positive things you can do is to seek out other mothers who are in the same boat. This shouldn't be too difficult, as you are almost bound to come into contact with lots of other pregnant mums at your local antenatal clinic. If you can discuss the question of weight in pregnancy with other mothers, you will be able to give each other moral support and compare and exchange your hopes and anxieties. It helps to know that other women are having the same difficulties as yourself, and sharing the problem with others is beneficial to all parties. Talking it through may give you more incentive to keep within the acceptable limits.

Most visits to antenatal clinics involve a certain amount of hanging around and sitting in waiting rooms, so there is a good opportunity to talk to other mothers-to-be. Most of us have very similar anxieties about pregnancy and childbirth, and discussing the things that worry you with other expectant mums is a very good way of working things through in your mind and sorting out your own difficulties. Naturally this goes for all aspects of pregnancy, not just the particular problem of coping with the weight you are gaining.

We in Britain are often accused of suffering from a 'national disease' which involves withdrawing from contact with each other in public places, avoiding eye-to-eye contact with strangers (in trains for instance), keeping very much to ourselves in places like waiting rooms, and being generally unsociable and over-polite to the point of negligence. There is probably a lot of truth in this – let's take, for example, our visits to the dentist or the doctor. We all sit there in silence, reprimanding the children if they dare to make a noise, refusing to look directly at other people in the waiting room, hiding behind magazines. Wouldn't it be much nicer if we all talked to each other instead? Wouldn't it be much better if we said something to one another occasionally and took a bit of an interest in each other? There must be something we all have in common, even if it's only sharing the particular dentist or doctor we happen to be visiting.

New motherhood can be a very lonely occupation. This may especially be so if you have given up an active job, perhaps the sort of job where you have been used to being surrounded by other people all day long. It is very important to have contact with other mothers in your area, or to keep up your old friendships at work. The thought of being pregnant for the first time, overweight, and suddenly cut off from work colleagues can be very depressing, and unfortunately some women tend to eat for compensation. Try to avoid this at all costs – instead, seek out other women who are in a similar situation and make an effort to talk to them throughout the course of your pregnancy. Talk to them (and also listen to them – it works both ways) about anything that particularly worries you, for example losing your figure or giving up your job. Everybody has some worries and misgivings about pregnancy, and a first pregnancy confronts you with a myriad of new feelings and sensations and a great deal of previously unknown territory to cover.

Pregnancy and Diet

If you are one of those people who are prone to being overweight and are now pregnant, try to keep an accurate account of your weight gain throughout your pregnancy. This will be done for you at your antenatal clinic, but to begin with you will only visit the clinic once a month. Make a weekly check yourself and keep a chart of your progress, starting as soon as you know you are pregnant. Then you will be able to judge for yourself whether you are managing satisfactorily or whether you are gaining weight too fast and need to take extra care. If you keep within the weight gain limits of 10 lb during the first five months and up to 20 lb during the last four months (26–30 lb altogether), you will be able to congratulate yourself on a job well done and enjoy your pregnancy without worrying. If, however, you find you are gaining weight too quickly from the start, place your weight chart on a prominent wall in the kitchen as an added incentive to refrain from culinary over-indulgence. In order to succeed you must want to help yourself. Don't kid yourself that being overweight doesn't matter, and believe and understand that it's up to *you* to look after yourself during your pregnancy, for your own sake and for the sake of your baby.

2

Good Nutrition in Pregnancy

What is good nutrition? In order to answer that question it is necessary to understand something of how the body works. Our bodies have certain basic requirements concerning the type of fuel we pump into our digestive systems. We all need a certain amount of protein, a particular quantity of carbohydrate, some fats, various mixtures of vitamins and minerals, adequate roughage, with a few trace elements thrown in, to make our bodies perform at the height of their potential. Good nutrition is the art of balancing the intake of all these bits and pieces throughout each day so that we receive all the relevant elements we need for our bodies to function normally and correctly. Usually this balance is fairly easily arrived at just by ensuring a varied, adventurous diet. In pregnancy, however, certain changes in nutritional requirements occur, and although these are only slight changes they are nevertheless very important for the development of the baby and the continued smooth-running effectiveness of the mother's body.

There is no doubt that a pregnant woman needs more to eat when she is carrying her child, but this should not become an excuse to over-eat. As well as generally needing more calories (see p. 20), specific extra nutrients are required for particular needs. A growing baby inside the womb is formed in its entirety from the food eaten by the mother. The nutrients in the food are absorbed into the mother's bloodstream in the normal way, then passed on to the baby through the placenta and umbilical cord. Soon after conception, while the embryo is still very tiny indeed and doesn't have enormous nutritional needs, much of the extra food the mother eats goes to provide nutrients for the production of the placenta and umbilical cord themselves. As the baby grows in size, so does the placenta, in order to cope with the increasing flow of nutrients from the mother to the baby. Some of the baby's waste is also passed back through the placenta into the mother's system so that she can filter it and excrete it along with her own waste. If the pregnant mother doesn't eat enough food to satisfy her own and her baby's needs, it will be the mother who suffers at first, because the baby will automatically extract the nutrients it needs from the stores in the mother's body. Energy is stored in the mother in the form of fat, iron is stored in the liver, and most vitamins and minerals are also stored in the body. If the mother's diet before pregnancy was not adequate for her own needs then some of these stores may already be exhausted at the time she conceives, and if throughout pregnancy the mother still does not eat adequately and correctly, mother and baby could *both* suffer from lack of the necessary nutrients, leading to abnormalities of function and growth. Some nutrients, such as Vitamin C, cannot be stored in the body at all, so it is very important indeed for the mother to eat foods containing these every day.

In order to be sure that you are combining the right sort of foods for a nutritious diet, it is a good idea to have a basic knowledge of how nutrition and digestion work. Included in this chapter are descriptions of the various different categories of nutrients in food, and a list of which foods contain them. There is also an explanation of why each category is necessary, and this is followed by a discussion of how dietary needs change more precisely in pregnancy and how to allow for this in your diet.

Protein

Protein can be used in three major ways in the body. Firstly, protein is needed for the repair of old, worn-out cells in your existing body, for the act of regeneration. Secondly, protein is vital in the process which enables completely new tissues to be formed, as in pregnancy. Thirdly, any extra protein taken into the body which is not needed directly for the first two processes can be turned into glucose and used to provide energy.

The way in which proteins are chemically made up is very complicated. Basically, however, proteins are constructed from amino acids and are found only in living things, in other words, animals and plants. *All* proteins contain varying amounts of carbon, oxygen, hydrogen and nitrogen, while some proteins also contain smaller amounts of other elements such as phosphorus or sulphur. Different proteins are made up from different combinations of the twenty-two individual amino acids. There are eight so-called 'essential' amino acids, and these must form part of our diet because they cannot be manufactured in the body. Foods containing all these essential amino acids are known as foods containing 'complete' proteins. The other fourteen amino acids are called 'non-essential' because they can be manufactured in the body by combining certain left-over bits and pieces. Foods containing non-essential amino acids and lacking any of the essential ones are known as foods containing 'incomplete' proteins. Animal protein is very like the protein in our own bodies in structure and is therefore usually complete protein. Vegetable protein is noticeably different in structure and is therefore generally incomplete protein, because it is usually lacking in one or more of the essential amino acids, which cannot be manufactured. However, this doesn't necessarily make vegetable protein of less value in the human diet than meat, because a good variety of vegetable protein each day can provide all the essential amino acids when eaten and digested together. A certain essential amino acid lacking in wheat, for instance, can be made up for by eating peanuts, which may include it. One vegetable, however, breaks all the rules because it is a complete protein like that of animals, containing all the eight essential amino acids. This vegetable is, of course, the soya bean, and it is certainly a very valuable bean indeed for those who prefer not to eat any meat or animal products in their diet.

Many parts of our bodies are made up and built from

proteins, including the most important ones such as the heart, lungs and brain. The number of organs in the body which are made from protein shows how the twenty-two amino acids can be strung together in many ways to form different kinds of protein. Blood, nerves and lymph are made from protein, as are muscles, hair, skin, teeth, eyes, nails, tendons and ligaments. Enzymes and hormones are also made from protein.

Amino acids themselves do not have the ability to be stored in our bodies, but any that are left over from the process of building and repairing are not wasted – they are taken to the liver where they are turned into glucose, which can be used for energy.

Which foods can we eat to ensure that we are getting enough protein into our systems? No one food is made purely from one type of nutrient (with the exception of some fats), so there is no food which consists of pure protein. Some foods have a high level of protein in them, and not much else besides, while other foods have an appreciable amount of protein coupled with a fair amount of something else, quite often starch, as in peas and beans.

FIG. 8. Protein chart.

High level protein foods (complete proteins)	Medium level protein foods (incomplete proteins)
Meat	**Pulses**
Pork	Red kidney beans
Lamb	Blackeye beans
Beef	Mung beans
Bacon	Chickpeas
Ham	Lentils
Veal	Haricot beans
Rabbit	Butter beans
	Aduki beans
Offal	Peas
Liver	
Heart	**Nuts and seeds**
Kidney	Almonds
	Walnuts

Good Nutrition in Pregnancy

High level protein foods (complete proteins)	Medium level protein foods (incomplete proteins)
Fish	**Nuts and seeds**
Cod	Brazil nuts
Plaice	Peanuts
Mackerel	Cashew nuts
Tuna	Sunflower seeds
Salmon	Sesame seeds
Sardines	
Herring	**Cereals**
Kippers	Wheat (whole)
Pilchards	Rye
Crab	Barley
Lobster	Brown rice
All shellfish	Oats
	Millet
Fowl	Maize
Chicken	
Turkey	
Pheasant	
Duck	
Goose	
Other wild game birds	
Eggs of all sorts	
Dairy products	
Milk	
Cheese	
Yogurt	
Buttermilk	
Pulses	
Soya beans	

Protein in pregnancy

As we have already seen, one of the most important functions of protein in the body is building new tissues. Pregnancy is an obvious example of this. During pregnancy a vast amount of extra protein is required to build not only the baby itself, but also all the supportive systems that nurture it inside the womb, such as the placenta, umbilical cord and enlarged, thickened uterus. The volume of blood in the mother's body increases, and there are also big fluctuations in the levels of hormones. A moderately active woman who is not pregnant has a minimum protein requirement of 38 g per day, while the recommended protein requirement for a pregnant woman is 60 g per day. This extra 22 g per day adds up over the whole nine months of pregnancy to over 6 kg. (While 60 g per day is the recommended intake of protein for a pregnant woman, it should be stressed that the absolute minimum she can get away with is 44 g per day.) A woman who is breastfeeding needs even more protein than during pregnancy, in order to produce enough milk to satisfy her baby. The recommended protein requirement for a breast-feeding mother is 68 g per day.

Carbohydrates

Carbohydrates are used by the body in two distinct ways. Firstly they provide energy for the body to use for activity, and secondly they can be turned into a store of latent energy which can be called on in the event of a shortage of fresh energy foods in the diet later on. The term *carbohydrate* covers three main areas of food – sugars, starches and fibre. All these groups are based on glucose, which is the basic carbohydrate unit.

Sugars. There are several different sugars, each of which is slightly different chemically. Glucose and fructose are simple sugars, and sucrose, maltose and lactose are more complex sugars. All digestible carbohydrate is broken down into glucose, which is the simplest, most basic unit of sugar, before being absorbed into the blood and then distributed to cells in the body to be used for energy.

Starches. Starches are more complex chemical structures, and have to be broken down into glucose again before they can be absorbed into the blood stream. Most cereals contain quite a lot of starch, as do certain root vegetables.

Fibre. The fibrous parts of vegetables, cereals and fruits are made from cellulose, which is an even more complex structure than starch and is also made from glucose. Humans cannot digest fibre at all, but it is necessary in the diet to provide bulk or roughage which promotes good digestion, stops constipation, and helps combat certain 'modern' diseases whose causes are linked to too much over-refined food in the diet, such as cancer of the colon.

Carbohydrate is needed in the diet to provide energy in several different ways. In the first place, energy is needed for direct physical activity such as walking or running. This sort of activity is called 'voluntary', because we choose to do it of our own free will. Due to the complex workings of our bodies there is another sort of activity which is called 'involuntary' action. This is the activity of certain organs inside our bodies, for example the heart and lungs, and this type of activity takes place without us even thinking about it and is therefore involuntary. Energy is also needed to bring about all the chemical reactions and activities, known as metabolism, that take place constantly in our bodies. Lastly, we need energy to keep us warm, so that we maintain an average body temperature however cold it is outside.

If we eat too much carbohydrate it can be turned into glycogen and stored in the liver and muscles, or it can be turned into fat and stored in the tissues as a layer of fat under the skin, forming a reservoir of energy that can be called on when fresh food is scarce.

These days it is important to distinguish between the different qualities of carbohydrate foods available. A great deal of *refined* carbohydrate is on sale in the form of white flour and white sugar, and is present in large amounts in many commercially produced food products. These refined carbohydrates are not of such good nutritional value as the unrefined, natural kind, which are found, for example, in wholewheat flour or wholewheat bread and naturally sweet foods like honey and sweet-tasting fruits. Refined carbohydrate foods lack fibre or cellulose, which is an extremely important part of our diet, especially during pregnancy. The reasons for its importance are discussed at greater length in Chapter 4, which concerns methods of changing your diet for the better, and in Chapter 6, which discusses some of the common ailments and discomforts of pregnancy which can be relieved by changes in the diet.

FIG. 9. *Carbohydrate chart.*

Sugar	Starch		Fibre
All processed sugars (sucrose)	*All cereals*	*All pulses*	All foods in the starches column of the carbohydrate chart, in their natural state, i.e. wholewheat flour, wholewheat bread, wholewheat pasta, brown rice
Syrup	Wheat	Red kidney beans	
Honey	Rye	Blackeye beans	
Molasses	Barley	Mung beans	
Maple syrup	Rice	Chickpeas	
Malt extract	Oats	Lentils	
Glucose	Millet	Haricot beans	
	Maize	Butter beans	
Fresh and dried fruit (fructose)	*Cereal products*	Aduki beans	
	Bread	Peas	
Milk and all dairy products (lactose)	Crispbread	Soya beans	
	Spaghetti and all types of pasta	*Vegetables*	Skins and fibrous parts of beans, vegetables and fruits
	Pastry	Potatoes	
	Oatmeal		
	Tapioca		Bran
	Semolina		

Carbohydrate in pregnancy

Pregnancy is a physically demanding time for most women and can be a tiring experience. Many women find that their energy levels are low at this time, and for this reason it is important to make sure that enough carbohydrate foods are eaten. Extra energy is needed during pregnancy not only to help carry around the extra 2 stone in weight which you can expect to gain by the end of the 9 months, but also to cope with the baby's metabolism as well as your own. During pregnancy you need to build up a 'store' of energy inside you in the form of a layer of fat, which you can draw on during the physically draining activity of childbirth and to produce milk for the baby in the days immediately following delivery. This extra fat should amount to about 4 or 5 lb.

Fats

Fat is needed in the body for several reasons. There is a layer of fat in the tissues underneath the skin, which protects the body from cold and helps to maintain the body temperature of the organs beneath it. This is called 'subcutaneous' fat. Fat is also needed right inside our bodies, where it wraps itself round some of the major organs to protect them and help hold them in place. This fat acts as a sort of shock absorber, keeping the different organs separate and helping to prevent them banging against each other during movement of the body. Even more important than this is the function which fat has in relation to some vitamins. Vitamin A, Vitamin D and Vitamin E can only be absorbed into the body with the aid of fat in the diet; they are called 'fat-soluble' vitamins and are essential for health. Lastly, different fats are made up from different combinations of fatty acids, and a few of these in particular are called 'essential' fatty acids because they are essential for health. While most of the fat the body needs can be manufactured inside the body from carbohydrates, these cannot, so they need to be included in the diet.

Fat is the most concentrated form of energy in food there is. This is not surprising when we consider that animals, and some plants too, rely on fat as a store of energy, an insurance against lack of food later. Evolution always takes the most simple, compact, thrifty path, so this store of energy in the form of fat is bound to be highly concentrated, efficient and economical.

Some of the fat which is stored in animals is clearly evident when the animal is slaughtered and used for food, for example the layer of fat surrounding the edge of a slice of ham, or the streaks of fat in streaky bacon. This type of fat is said to be 'visible', because it can easily be seen. Other fats, however, are 'invisible', because they are mixed in with other parts of the food and are less obvious; for example, the extra fat in muscle tissue in the lean parts of a cut of meat, the fat in the flesh of certain oily fish, or the high level of fat which is found in most nuts and seeds. All types of fat are made up from fatty acids. There are many different kinds of fatty acids, and they can combine together in a variety of ways to produce a large number of different types of fats. Fats are very high in calories indeed, having about 225 per 1 oz of fat, so while a small amount of fat is essential in the diet, care should be taken not to eat too much.

The difference between fats and oils

Most people realize that 'oil' is a term used for fat in a liquid state, but understanding why some fats are liquid and some solid is more complicated. The answer lies in the type of fatty acids that go to make up a fat or an oil. Most people will have heard of the terms 'saturated' and 'polyunsaturated' in relation to butter and margarines. Most fats contain both saturated and polyunsaturated fatty acids, but in different proportions. A fat containing larger quantities of saturated fatty acids is more likely to be solid, while a fat which contains more polyunsaturated fatty acids is more likely to be liquid. Thus most polyunsaturated fats are liquid oils.

Saturated fatty acids have a particular chemical structure which means they won't 'go off' or go rotten in a normal atmosphere, while polyunsaturated fatty acids have a different structure which means that they will react chemically and go rancid when they come into contact with the air. This is why all the artificially hardened margarines made with polyunsaturated vegetable oils contain large amounts of preservatives, to give them a longer shelf life in the shops. The best quality vegetable oils are those which are cold-pressed. This means that the oil is extracted from the plant or seed by the simple method of pressing heavy weights on them, without using heat (see p. 92).

Cholesterol

There has been a great deal of discussion over the past few years about the role played by cholesterol in relation to certain diseases of the heart and the occurrence of heart attacks in men. Cholesterol is most commonly found in animal products, and is particularly high in animal fats and eggs. If you are worried about the amount of cholesterol in your family's diet, you can easily put your mind at rest by cutting down on some of the animal fats you use in your cooking, such as lard, suet or dripping, and substituting vegetable oils, which contain no cholesterol at all. It is certainly not necessary to cut out animal fats altogether,

FIG. 10. Fat chart.

Visible fats	Invisible fats
Butter	Milk
Lard	Cheese
Suet	Eggs
Dripping	Cream
Margarine	Mayonnaise
Bacon fat	Salad dressings
Fat surrounding cuts of meat	Unseen fat in all lean meats and fowl
Olive oil	All processed meat products
Almond oil	Herrings
Soya bean oil	Salmon
Corn oil	Sardines
Sunflower oil	Mackerel
Sesame seed oil	Pilchards
Peanut oil	Tuna fish
	All nuts and seeds
	Chocolate
	Pastry
	Biscuits
	Cakes

unless you are particularly at risk, but a general aim to use more vegetable oils instead of animal fats is probably a good idea.

Fats in pregnancy

A varied diet will contain enough fats and oils to supply the body with the quantity of fat it needs, so as long as you continue to follow a varied diet in pregnancy you will have nothing to worry about. The only problem you may have is eating *too much* fat, since so much of it is invisible in our diet. Take care to avoid eating too much fat while you are pregnant by cutting down on fried foods and grilling or baking instead.

Vitamins

Each vitamin has a different role to play in keeping our bodies healthy, but basically they all form an important part of the process by which food is used to build and maintain our bodies. Vitamins assist the body in using and absorbing the other nutrients from our food. If we ate food that was totally lacking in vitamins, our bodies would not be able to use the energy the food provided. Each vitamin has a specialized job to do.

Vitamins fall into two main categories, those which are 'fat-soluble' and those which are 'water-soluble'. If too large a quantity of water-soluble vitamins is taken in no harm is done, because any excess is excreted by the body. Too large a quantity of fat-soluble vitamins, however, is not so easily dealt with, as they can accumulate in the body and can be harmful, so care should be taken not to overdo your intake of fat-soluble vitamins through taking too many vitamin pills. If your diet is reasonably varied and you are aware of your basic nutritional needs, it is unlikely that you will normally need a supplement of vitamins of any sort. Pregnancy, however, does necessitate a slightly larger intake of certain vitamins, such as folic acid (see p. 41).

FAT-SOLUBLE VITAMINS	WATER-SOLUBLE VITAMINS
Vitamin A	Vitamin B1 (thiamin)
Vitamin D	Vitamin B2 (riboflavin)
Vitamin E	Vitamin B6 (pyridoxine)
Vitamin K	Nicotinic acid (niacin)
	Biotin
	Pantothenic acid
	Folic acid
	Vitamin C

N.B. Vitamin B12 is not water-soluble but is absorbed in the small intestine by another process.

Fat-soluble vitamins

VITAMIN A. This is the vitamin which is concerned with the eyes, especially with the ability to see well in bad light. It is also associated with keeping all the mucous membranes in the body healthy, and has some effect on the skin. Particularly large amounts of Vitamin A can be found naturally in fish liver (hence cod liver oil), and in the flesh of other fatty fish such as herring, salmon, sardines and tuna. It is also found in animal livers and kidneys, as well as in eggs and most dairy produce. All synthetically produced margarines must include added Vitamin A by law, as do certain breakfast cereals. Vitamin A can also be manufactured inside the body from carotene, which is the orange colouring found in carrots and other orange or yellow fruits and vegetables.

VITAMIN D. Vitamin D and calcium go hand in hand, because calcium cannot be absorbed into the body unless Vitamin D accompanies it in the intestines. For this reason it is a particularly important vitamin for young children, who need lots of calcium to grow healthy bones and teeth, and also for pregnant mothers, who need to pass on both calcium and Vitamin D via the placenta to the baby in the womb so that its bones can form properly. It is also important for breastfeeding mothers to get enough Vitamin D, so that the calcium the baby gets through its mother's milk can be put to good use. Vitamin D can be found in the same foods as Vitamin A, including fatty fish like salmon and tuna, dairy products and margarine. It can also be derived from the action of sunlight on the skin (see 'Fresh air', pp. 76–7).

VITAMIN E. This vitamin is often said to be closely associated with fertility, though this has yet to be completely proven as far as humans are concerned. Women who have trouble conceiving would do better to follow the pre-conception diet given in Chapter 4 for several months and ask the advice of their doctors, instead of relying on taking extra Vitamin E. Most diets contain plenty of Vitamin E anyway, as it is fairly widespread in food, so extra supplements of it should not need to be taken except in very unusual circumstances. Vitamin E is found in very small quantities in most foods, but good sources are all fats and oils, wheatgerm, cereals and eggs.

VITAMIN K. This vitamin has to do with the ability of blood to clot properly. You are unlikely to suffer from a lack of Vitamin K because it is found in many different foods, and also because it can be made by the body itself. When a deficiency does occur it is usually in small babies, as the result of a problem in the transference of the vitamin to the baby from the mother. Vitamin K is prolific in all green vegetables, especially spring greens, spinach, cauliflower, cabbage and peas. It is also found in cereals.

Water-soluble vitamins

Water-soluble vitamins dissolve in water and are therefore easily excreted in the urine. This means that it is important to include a regular supply of foods containing these vitamins in the diet, especially during pregnancy, as they cannot be stored for any length of time in the body.

VITAMIN B1 (THIAMIN), VITAMIN B2 (RIBOFLAVIN), and NICOTINIC ACID (NIACIN). These three vitamins are grouped together because they have a very similar job to do – each is responsible in a slightly different way for activating the release of a regular, non-stop supply of energy for the body from carbohydrate. Vitamin B1 is found in many different foods, but especially in offal, milk, eggs, wholegrain cereals, fruit and vegetables. Vitamin B2 is also found in a great variety of foods, but there is an especially high quantity in fresh milk. Nicotinic acid is found in meat, flour and some vegetables, but it can also be manufactured in the body from nutrients found in milk and eggs.

VITAMIN B6 (PYRIDOXINE). This vitamin is involved in the process by which protein is released into the body in a form which can be used for building and repairing body tissues. It is a good idea to ensure that you get plenty of this vitamin during pregnancy, as it is also responsible for part of the process of making haemoglobin in the blood. All vitamins connected with manufacturing blood are very important in pregnancy, not only to increase the volume of blood in the mother's body so that she can cope with the baby's metabolism as well as her own, but also to form the baby's blood itself. Vitamin B6 is found in many foods, including meat, fish, eggs and wholegrain cereals.

BIOTIN. This is necessary so that the body can use fat, and is found in egg yolk, offal and cereals.

PANTOTHENIC ACID. This is used in the process by which both fat and carbohydrate are released for energy. It is found in meat and in a wide variety of vegetables and cereals.

FOLIC ACID. This is especially important for pregnant women, and for babies who are born prematurely, because it is involved in the process of making new blood, particularly new red blood cells. Because the need for adequate folic acid is so acute in pregnancy, it used to be routinely prescribed by doctors along with extra iron as soon as it was discovered that a woman was pregnant. Now it seems that medical opinion is divided on whether or not every pregnant woman needs extra folic acid and iron as a matter of course, and some doctors think it necessary to prescribe it only for those women who are obviously at risk of not getting the quantity they need. If you are not offered any when you become pregnant, make sure you eat plenty of the foods that are rich in folic acid to ensure an adequate natural supply, particularly in early pregnancy when the need is greatest. Folic acid is found naturally in offal and in raw, green vegetables. It must be emphasized, however, that it is very easily destroyed by cooking, so it is important to eat plenty of salads using leafy, green vegetables, and only to lightly cook or steam other green vegetables.

VITAMIN C (ASCORBIC ACID). This is probably the best-known vitamin of all, and is essential for keeping connective tissue in the body healthy. Since we cannot store Vitamin C in the body we need to ensure that we eat a fresh supply every day, especially in pregnancy. Complete lack of Vitamin C in the diet causes scurvy and bleeding gums. Again, Vitamin C is one of those vitamins which is easily destroyed by cooking, so it is essential to get a supply from fresh, uncooked foods, or to take a supplement. Vitamin C can be found in fruit and vegetables, especially blackcurrants, rosehips, lemons, oranges, strawberries, cabbage, cauliflower, Brussels sprouts and potatoes.

VITAMIN B12. This is neither a water-soluble vitamin nor a fat-soluble one, but is absorbed into the body by a complex system involving certain gastric juices. It is used in conjunction with folic acid, and is needed by cells which divide very quickly, such as bone marrow cells which turn into blood. Without any Vitamin B12 you would become anaemic. Vitamin B12 is not found in any plants at all (with the exception of yeast), but only in animal foods, particularly in meat and offal (especially liver). Vegetarians are at risk of not getting enough Vitamin B12 because they eat no meat, although small amounts are found in milk, cheese, eggs and yeast extract. Pregnant mothers who are also vegetarians are particularly at risk.

Minerals

Minerals are inorganic elements which are needed by the body for various activities, and seven of them are needed in fairly large quantities. The rest are only needed in very minute amounts – these are called trace elements.

IRON. The way that iron works in the body is fairly complicated, but basically it is a major constituent of haemoglobin in the blood, which is responsible for distributing the oxygen which is breathed into the lungs to all the cells in the body which need it. This is a very important function, and an adequate supply of iron is especially important during pregnancy. Women of childbearing age often lose a lot of blood during menstruation, and the iron that is lost in this way is usually replaced by iron-rich foods in the diet. However, if the monthly loss of blood is very heavy there may not be enough iron in the diet to replace that lost, which means that the body must use up its store of iron in the liver, and the eventual result will be anaemia. Anaemia need not be a very serious complaint if it is treated quickly. The usual symptoms of anaemia include general lack of energy, listlessness and a general feeling of tiredness, none of which is too distressing to begin with. However, it is easy for these symptoms to be wrongly attributed to other factors, such as pregnancy itself, or depression, so that the anaemia may often be fairly advanced before it is diagnosed correctly. For this reason it is a good idea to make sure you are getting plenty of iron before you conceive. If you do not, you risk starting your pregnancy with dangerously low levels of iron in your blood system, and these could drop even lower as the pregnancy continues.

A pregnant woman needs a greater volume of blood than normal to cope with the growth and metabolism of the baby inside her. The baby's blood also has to be manufactured, using nutrients from the mother, and there must be a big enough store of extra blood to ensure that if any is lost during the birth of the child this will not be detrimental to the mother. Also, a store of iron has to be built up in the baby's own liver during its nine months in the womb, because its main source of food for the first six months or so after its birth, milk, does not contain a great amount of iron. At the same time it is important that a breastfeeding mother has an adequate supply of iron after the birth, because the small amount of iron which is contained in breast milk will always be maintained, despite the fact that the mother's own supply may be low. For all these reasons it used to be routine for doctors in this country to prescribe extra iron in tablet form as soon as a woman discovered that she was pregnant. Some doctors, however, do not now consider this to be necessary, and will not prescribe extra iron as a matter of course. To be on the safe side, make sure you eat plenty of iron-rich foods or buy your own iron supplement from a chemist. Iron can be found in offal (especially liver), red meat, eggs, cereals and green vegetables. However, not all the iron in your food is readily absorbed into your blood, so the recommended intakes are higher than those actually needed.

CALCIUM. This is another very important mineral in the diet, as it is a major constituent of bones and teeth. A baby's bones are formed quite early in pregnancy, so a good supply of calcium is essential from the start. The baby will take all the calcium it needs from its mother's body regardless of the effect on her health, so it is important for the mother to have enough, not so much for the baby's sake as for her own. In women who have had many pregnancies where their calcium intake has been insufficient, the result is decalcified bones which are brittle and break easily. Breastfeeding mothers also need plenty of calcium in their diet, because so much calcium goes into the production of milk for the baby. We have seen that not all the iron that is eaten in the diet is absorbed into the body, and it is the same with calcium. Only a quarter of the calcium eaten is absorbed, and the rest is lost through excretion. Even less calcium would be absorbed if it were not for Vitamin D, which acts in conjunction with calcium to utilize it more efficiently in the body. Young children who do not get enough calcium suffer from rickets, the symptoms of which are deformed bones and stunted growth. Calcium is found in milk, cheese, bread, and some vegetables, for example watercress and cabbage, and some can also be found in the soft bones of tinned fish such as salmon, pilchards and sardines.

PHOSPHORUS. Like calcium, this important mineral is used for making strong bones and teeth. It is also responsible for using and releasing energy from food. It is found in a great variety of foods, so it is unlikely that anyone will suffer from a lack of it in this country. Foods containing large quantities of phosphorus include dairy produce, eggs, meat, fish, peanuts and wholewheat bread.

MAGNESIUM. This is another mineral necessary for forming bones, and is also involved with the work of some enzymes. The main sources of magnesium are green vegetables, but it can also be found in smaller quantities in many other foods.

POTASSIUM. This is involved with the liquids in cells, and is found in meat, vegetables and milk.

CHLORINE and SODIUM. These two go together because when combined they make salt, which is needed in the body to help maintain the balance of water. Salt is not found in large quantities in natural, unprocessed foods, but is often added during the preparation of food. Small babies should not be given salt in their diet because, unlike adults, they are unable to get rid of any excess through the kidneys.

Trace elements

Trace elements are needed by the body in tiny quantities only, but they are nevertheless essential to good health. They are all usually adequately supplied by eating a good variety of different foods, so supplements are unlikely to be necessary. In fact it has been found that too large a quantity of some of these trace elements, for example, copper, can be poisonous.

IODINE. This is one of the components of the hormones manufactured by the thyroid gland. It is found in seawater fish and shellfish, and also in vegetables grown in soil with a high iodine content. It is also possible to buy iodized salt which can be used instead of plain table salt.

ZINC. This is involved in the working of certain enzymes, and can be found in many different categories of foods.

FLUORINE. This is an important element in the formation of bones and teeth, especially in children. In some areas it occurs naturally in drinking water, while in others it is synthetically added to the water supply. It is also found in tea and fish, and is sometimes given to children in tablet form.

MANGANESE. This element is involved in the action of enzymes and is found in tea, wholegrain cereals, nuts and spices.

COPPER. This is another trace element involved in the action of enzymes, this time in particular with the production of haemoglobin. It is found in a variety of foods.

COBALT. This is part of the structure of Vitamin B12, and is thus concerned with the production of red blood cells. Cobalt is found in all animal products.

Fibre

Fibre is important in the diet because it adds bulk to the faeces, thus aiding the passage of waste through the intestines. The whole process of digestion from one end to the other usually takes between one and three days if a healthy diet is eaten, but with a diet that is very low in fibre, digestion can take up to a week. During pregnancy it is especially important to make sure that there is enough fibre in the diet, because at this time the whole process of digestion slows down. This digestive sluggishness is due in particular to extra progesterone in the blood during pregnancy, which has the effect of lowering the muscle tone of the digestive organs, resulting in the food staying longer in the intestines and leading eventually to constipation. This can be counteracted by eating more fibre, because, unlike other food, fibre is not digested in the stomach but passes straight through; by the time it reaches the gut it will have absorbed a lot of extra water, thus providing more bulk in the stools and making them softer and easier to get rid of. Fibre is made of cellulose, which basically is the structure of the cell walls of plants. Wholefoods and healthfoods, or foods which are in their whole, natural state, contain their full quota of fibre, which many processed foods lack. The act of 'processing' or 'refining' plant foods usually involves stripping away the cellulose or fibrous parts of the food, leaving the rest in a concentrated, fibreless state. Examples are wholewheat flour and its processed counterpart white flour, or brown rice and its processed counterpart white rice. In order to get adequate supplies of fibre, use plant foods that are in as nearly natural a state as possible. Use wholewheat flour, pasta, bread and pastry, look out for brown rice, and eat more whole grains such as muesli or porridge. Add wheat bran to soups and stews or sprinkle it on your breakfast cereal. Pulses (dried peas and beans), wholegrain cereals, dried fruits, fresh fruit and fresh vegetables are all good sources of fibre.

There are other ways in which you can increase your fibre intake, in particular by taking care how you cook your food. Although fibre cannot be digested by the human body, it can be broken down by boiling and over-cooking and sometimes by quick freezing. So make an effort to use fresh, uncooked vegetables and fruit, and if you must cook them, do so gently and for a short time only. Don't boil your vegetables to a mush, but cook them just enough to make them palatable yet still slightly crunchy. This way you will retain most of the fibre in a state in which your body can use it. Leave the skins on potatoes and other root vegetables, and when you eat an apple eat the core as well. Foods that are full of fibre need more chewing, and this should also help to satisfy your increased appetite during pregnancy, so that you won't put on too much weight.

However, there is one very important fact to remember when you are adding more fibre to your diet during pregnancy: extra fibre not only increases the rate at which food passes through the digestive system, it also means that the body has less time to extract the nutrients it needs from the food. This is particularly true with calcium. The absorption of calcium is greatly reduced when more fibre is eaten, and calcium is one of the very important minerals needed by the body during pregnancy (see pp. 44–5). So if you are going to make a conscious effort to increase your fibre intake during pregnancy, make sure that you also increase your calcium intake to allow for the reduced absorption.

Water

The human body can survive for quite a long time without food, because of the stores of fat which can be drawn on in an emergency, but without water the body will die within a few days, as excessive dehydration makes it impossible for it to carry out the metabolic processes necessary for life. Water is used by the body in many different ways – in fact over half the body is made of water. All the cells of the soft tissues and organs in the body contain a watery liquid called the 'intercellular fluid'. Liquid outside the cells is called the 'extracellular fluid', and these two watery liquids are the medium through which most of the nutrients are taken from food and used by the body in the cells. The nutrients are moved around the body by the blood, which also has a high water content.

We take water into our bodies in various ways, and the most obvious of these is drinking. We drink when we are thirsty, but we also take water into our bodies when we eat, as most food contains some water. Some, for example juicy fruits or vegetables such as cucumber, contain a very large quantity of water indeed. Water is lost from the body in several different ways too. A lot of water is lost through urinating and in the faeces, but some is also lost through evaporation from the skin (sweating) and the lungs. This intake and loss of water is regulated by the kidneys so that the body ends up with the correct balance of liquid it needs. Certain medical conditions with symptoms of severe sweating or acute vomiting or diarrhoea can upset the balance, so that extra liquid needs to be taken. Pregnancy also increases the need for liquid, because you are taking in and losing water not only for yourself but also for the growing baby. Since during pregnancy the volume of blood in the mother's body increases and extra water is retained in the tissues, there will be a greater need for water at this time and you may need to consume extra liquid each day. (Don't forget, you won't necessarily need to *drink* all your liquids as you will get some from your food as well.) Mothers who choose to breastfeed their babies need an even greater supply of water in order to have enough liquid in their bodies to supply the milk, and it is a generally accepted habit to drink a glass of water every time you breastfeed your baby in order to replenish the liquid that has been taken from you.

The obvious drinks include water, tea, coffee, fruit and vegetable juices, herb teas, and milk. Foods containing large quantities of water include soups, stews, juicy fruits, vegetables and eggs. Try to keep away from sweetened drinks and fizzy 'cola' type drinks, because these will almost certainly contain a lot of sugar and will make you put on weight – they won't do your teeth any good either. If you really must drink this type of liquid, look out for the low calorie versions.

Suggested menus for one week

To help you visualize more easily the way in which natural foods can be incorporated into your diet, here is a suggested week's menus. Each day's menu adds up to 2,000 calories, which is the minimum you should allow yourself during the last two-thirds of your pregnancy. If you find you are still hungry at this level, and providing your weight gain is within the normal, expected limits, you may add up to another 400 calories maximum per day of extra food or drink, making your daily total 2,400.

Pregnancy and Diet

Breakfast
1 egg, boiled or poached
2 oz (55 g) wholemeal bread
¼ oz (7 g) butter
1 orange, approx. 6 oz (170 g)

¼ pint (140 ml) apple juice

Mid-morning snack
tea or coffee
1 fresh pear

Lunch
3 oz (85 g) Camembert or Brie cheese
2 oz (55 g) wholemeal bread
¼ oz (7 g) butter
mixed salad, made from equal quantities of lettuce, spring onions,
celery, red pepper, bean sprouts
1 oz (30 g) chutney

1 banana, approx. 6 oz (170 g)
1 small slice 2 oz (55 g) fruit cake (preferably sugar-free)

⅓ pint (200 ml) cold milk

Supper
4 oz (115 g) grilled liver
2 oz (55 g) grilled lean bacon
3 oz (85 g) boiled brown rice
3 oz (85 g) lightly boiled carrots
2 oz (55 g) lightly boiled peas

2 oz (55 g) dried apricots and 1 oz (30 g) sultanas, simmered together
in water

chamomile herb tea

Breakfast

2 oz (55 g) muesli (sugar-free)
¼ pint (140 ml) milk

¼ pint (140 ml) orange juice

Lunch

3 oz (85 g) sliced lean ham
¼ pint (140 ml) homemade onion sauce
4 oz (115 g) baked potato (eat skin too)
4 oz (115 g) steamed broccoli
2 oz (55 g) grilled mushrooms
1 grilled tomato

¼ pint (140 ml) plain yogurt
1 oz (30 g) chopped dates

tea or coffee

Supper

6 oz (170 g) quiche, made with wholemeal pastry
mixed salad, made from equal quantities of cucumber, tomato, raw
white cabbage, grated carrot
2 oz (55 g) sweetcorn

1 fresh peach

milk shake, made by whisking together ¼ pint (140 ml) milk, 1 raw
egg and 1 dessertspoon honey

Pregnancy and Diet

Breakfast

porridge made with 1 oz (30 g) porridge oats and ¼ pint (140 ml)
milk, topped with 1 oz (30 g) stewed dried fruit

1 oz (30 g) wholemeal bread
¼ oz (7 g) butter
1 oz (30 g) honey

¼ pint (140 ml) pineapple juice

Lunch

omelette made from 2 eggs, 1 oz (30 g) chopped onion, 1 oz (30 g)
cooked red kidney beans and 1 tablespoonful chopped fresh parsley,
and cooked in 1 dessertspoonful vegetable oil
salad made from equal quantities of bean sprouts, orange segments,
watercress

2 oz (55 g) mixed cashew nuts, almonds, walnuts
1 banana, approx. 6 oz (170 g)

¼ pint (140 ml) tomato juice

Supper

2 chicken drumsticks, baked or grilled
2 oz (55 g) broad beans
2 oz (55 g) grilled tomatoes
2 oz (55 g) sliced red and green peppers
¼ pint (140 ml) parsley sauce

4 oz (115 g) curd cheese, mixed with 1 dessertspoon honey and
topped with 4 oz (115 g) grapes

tea or coffee

THURSDAY

Breakfast

5 oz (140 g) kipper fillet
3 oz (85 g) cooked bulghur wheat
¼ oz (7 g) butter

¼ pint (140 ml) plain yogurt
¼ oz (7 g) sunflower seeds

tea or coffee

Lunch

8 oz (225 g) baked potato
1 oz (30 g) sliced lean ham
4 oz (115 g) cottage cheese
2 oz (55 g) raw cauliflower
lettuce, celery, French beans

fresh fruit salad made from ½ apple, ½ orange, ½ banana, 1 oz
(30 g) grapes
1 dessertspoonful honey

¼ pint (140 ml) apple juice

Supper

individual pizza (wholewheat)
mixed green salad made from green peppers, cucumber, chicory,
mustard and cress
2 oz (55 g) cooked beetroot

1 baked apple, stuffed with 2 oz (55 g) sultanas and 1 teaspoonful
honey

tea or coffee

Breakfast

2 oz (55 g) wholemeal roll
½ oz (15 g) butter
1 oz (30 g) tahini (sesame spread)

8 oz (225 g) slice melon
1 pear

¼ pint (140 ml) tomato juice

Mid morning
tea or coffee

Lunch

1 corn on the cob
½ oz (15 g) butter
2 oz (55 g) wholemeal bread
2 oz (55 g) sliced raw red cabbage, mixed with ½ oz (15 g) flaked
almonds

2 oz (55 g) peanuts and raisins

tea or coffee

Supper

6 oz (170 g) cod fillet
¼ pint (140 ml) parsley sauce
½ oz (15 g) pumpkin seeds
4 oz (115 g) boiled potatoes
2 oz (55 g) leeks
2 oz (55 g) courgettes
½ bunch watercress

1 slice fruit cake, 3 oz (85 g)

mint herb tea

Good Nutrition in Pregnancy

Breakfast

2 scrambled eggs, sprinkled with ½ oz (15 g) sesame seeds
2 oz (55 g) wholemeal bread
½ oz (15 g) butter

¼ pint (140 ml) hot milk, flavoured with ground cinnamon

Lunch

6 oz (170 g) mixed bean salad, made from red kidney beans,
chickpeas and soya beans
2 oz (55 g) grated raw carrot
2 oz (55 g) spinach
2 oz (55 g) turnip
4 oz (115 g) cooked potato, topped with 2 oz (55 g) plain yogurt

3 oz (55 g) (dry weight) dried mixed fruit and 1 fresh pear, stewed
in ¼ pint (140 ml) orange juice and sprinkled with ¼ oz (7 g)
desiccated coconut

Rose-hip herb tea

Supper

¼ sliced avocado
4 oz (115 g) cottage cheese
1 oz (30 g) sliced lean ham
salad made from onion rings, tomatoes, mushrooms, green pepper
1 oz (30 g) cooked peas
4 oz (115 g) cooked buckwheat grains

6 oz (170 g) brown rice pudding

tea or coffee

Breakfast

3 oz (85 g) mixed dried fruit, stewed in ¼ pint (140 ml) apple juice

1 poached egg
1 oz (30 g) wholemeal bread
½ oz (15 g) butter

tea or coffee

Lunch

4 oz (115 g) lean roast meat (beef, pork or lamb)
6 oz (170 g) baked potato
2 oz (55 g) each of cabbage, mushrooms, tomatoes, sprouts, sautéed
in 1 tablespoon vegetable oil
3 tablespoons thick gravy

1 oz (30 g) wholemeal bread spread with 1 oz (30 g) honey and
sprinkled with 1 teaspoon chopped mixed nuts

tea or coffee

Supper

4 oz (115 g) tuna fish (tinned in brine)
mixed green salad made from cucumber, lettuce, spring onions,
green peppers, and topped with 3 oz (85 g) plain yogurt
4 oz (115 g) cooked wholemeal macaroni

2 oz (55 g) mixed nuts and raisins

¼ pint (140 ml) hot milk, flavoured with a pinch of ground nutmeg
and allspice

3

Preconception Care

How your present lifestyle can affect your future family

What does it matter if you eat junk foods? Why should you bother to stop smoking now, when you may not be planning to start a family yet anyway? Why do you need to take stock of your eating habits and way of life long before you plan a pregnancy? The answers are simple. It can take up to six months to become really fit, and the fittest and healthiest babies are born to the fittest and healthiest mothers. Your body is the vessel in which your baby grows, it is the means by which your baby is nourished and grows mature enough for birth and independent life. Your body is responsible for producing the egg that grows into a new human being after penetration by the sperm. It is vital, then, that the egg itself is healthy and in the peak of condition, and a healthy mother is far more likely to produce a healthy egg. Naturally it is just as important for the sperm to be healthy and in good condition, so that when the egg and the sperm unite the fertilized ovum grows into as perfect a baby as possible. So a prospective father should take equal care to eat well, stop smoking and generally get fit all round before parenting any children.

Why does it take so long to get fit? Our bodies take time to adjust to new habits and to get the benefit of changing from bad habits to good. Traces of nicotine from cigarettes, alcohol from spirits or wine or beer, and hormones from contraceptive pills can stay in our bodies for quite a long time. To get the maximum benefit from discarding these we need to wait from three to six months, to be quite sure that the dangerous elements in them have left our bodies completely. It takes time for the body to build up stores of certain vitamins and minerals. It takes time for the body to eliminate the poisons that accumulate in our systems through eating junk foods with high levels of preservatives, colourings, artificial flavourings and additives. It also takes time for exercise to have a positive effect on the muscles and to build up stamina and strength in the body. All these things need to be done gradually, so it is important to give yourself plenty of time to make the changes in your diet and lifestyle that are guaranteed to maximize your chances of giving birth to a healthy baby. A great deal of benefit will be noticed after only three months if you persevere, but to be absolutely sure that you have done your very best for your baby it is advisable to give yourself six clear months of positive action in this way – this applies to both mother *and* father.

There are no hard and fast rules about preconceptual care. No one expects you to give up smoking and alcohol and to change your eating habits all in one go, so give yourself plenty of time. If you don't feel able to tackle all the ideas here at once, try just one or two to begin with. Take one step at a time and you will find it much easier. After a while it will become second nature to you and you will then be able to try the next step. For example, if you think you may be able to give up smoking but you just can't face doing without your daily dose of sugary confectionery (yes, sugar is addictive), then don't worry. Doing without cigarettes but still eating junk foods is better than continuing to do both, and vice versa. Just attempt whatever you feel you can cope with at the beginning and then gradually add the next item to your list. This way you will become fit and healthy gradually and it won't be too much of a shock to your system. Aim for the ideal by all means, but don't feel that you must reach it at any cost. Your state of mind is just as important as the state of your body! So don't overdo it, but take time to do it well.

No prospective parents relish the thought of having a damaged baby, handicapped mentally or physically, and many mothers-to-be try not to think about it too much in advance, telling themselves it can't happen to them. Yet year after year more damaged babies are born into the world, and this is a terrible shame when we know that there is something each of us can do in a positive way to help ensure healthy children. It is becoming increasingly clear in the medical world that many of these birth defects can be minimized or even eradicated altogether by careful preconceptual care of would-be parents. There are many different factors which affect the health of a growing foetus, but if it has a healthy environment in which to grow it stands a far greater chance of being healthy itself. It certainly cannot be said that *all* birth defects are preventable, but it is true to say that many can be avoided and the effects of others lessened by taking care in the months before you conceive. After conception, most of the baby's vital organs are formed within the first twelve weeks. Most of this important foetal development takes place in very early pregnancy, so by the time you discover that you are pregnant it is already too late to have any real effect on the vital early development and growth of the baby. This is why it is so important to take care of yourself and eat well during these first weeks of pregnancy and during the months before you conceive, in order to ensure that the egg and the sperm which join to form the baby are as healthy and fit as possible.

What you eat is obviously very important indeed, as the nutrients from the mother's blood are the raw materials which are used for building the baby. Eating the right food is *so* important that I have dedicated a whole chapter to the art of eating well. You have already read about your nutritional needs during pregnancy in Chapter 2. Chapter 4 will show you how to apply that knowledge to your choice of food, how to ensure that your diet is nutritionally sound and well balanced, how to cut down on junk foods and how to replace them with the correct alternatives. And don't forget that healthy eating is for fathers too.

But it is not only what you take in that is important during pregnancy, but also what you leave out. Bad habits such as smoking, excess alcohol, drugs and pollution can all affect the unborn child, and if you do away with or cut down on these things your unborn baby is bound to benefit and have a greater chance of being healthy. Certain medical conditions, age, sleep, exercise and weight all have a bearing on the unborn baby, and these considerations are described in the following pages. Don't leave it until it is too late – *start now*, before you conceive. (If you are already pregnant don't panic, just do as much as you can in the right direction by following the suggestions in this and the following chapter and you will still do yourself and your baby a lot of good.)

Not only will your baby get the benefit from the trouble you take, but so will you. You will feel better and look better, at a time when many women feel sick and rotten. Pregnancy can be tiring and exhausting, so look after yourself beforehand and you will have more strength and energy to draw on when you need it most.

Smoking

Smoking tobacco when you are *not* pregnant is a matter for your own conscience, as it is your own body you are endangering and we all have freedom of choice in such matters. If you *choose* to smoke, knowing the dangers and realizing the risks to your own life, then no one can really argue with you because it's *your* life and *your* choice. Smoking in pregnancy, however, is altogether different, because you are responsible not only for your own health but also for that of someone else, someone who cannot yet make any plea to you on their own behalf, but who nevertheless relies on you for their safety in the womb. Unlike some drugs which are prevented from reaching the baby because they are filtered out of the bloodstream, nicotine passes freely from mother to baby via the placenta. It is most unfair to force poisonous nicotine into the bloodstream of an unborn baby when you consider the effects it will undoubtedly have. It is damaging to the baby because it causes 'hypoxia' – this means that less oxygen reaches the baby through the placenta, thereby depriving it of some of the raw materials it needs in order to grow properly. It is well known that the babies of mothers who smoke are smaller than normal. They can be up to 7 oz lighter than babies born to mothers who do not smoke. Because of this they are prone to breathing difficulties immediately after delivery, and are also more likely to suffer from infections of various sorts. There is some evidence that children born to mothers who smoke go on suffering throughout childhood, as they continue to be weaker and less intelligent. Even at the age of seven or eight they may still be two or three months behind in reading and writing skills. We know for sure that babies who are exposed to nicotine in the womb are born smaller than normal, so it is possible that in these cases the placentas are also smaller and less efficient than normal, thereby depriving the foetus of nutrients as well as oxygen. If for some reason the placenta is not working properly anyway, smoking could be the decisive factor that could cause the death of the baby before it is born at all. Smoking is likely to increase the chance of a baby being stillborn or dying during the first few days after delivery. In the early months of pregnancy, spontaneous abortion or miscarriage is more likely. Mothers who are very heavy smokers run the risk of producing babies who suffer from cerebral palsy. Certain women are even more likely to encounter disaster if they continue to smoke, for example those who have high blood pressure, those who have previously had a stillbirth, those who have a history of previous miscarriages and those who encounter bleeding during pregnancy. So please don't take any more risks – for the sake of your children, if you are considering parenthood or are already pregnant, stop smoking now.

If you find it too hard to give up on your own, ask your doctor for advice and addresses of local organizations who can help and encourage you, or contact ASH, at 5–11 Mortimer Street, London, WIN 7RH. It is also very important for fathers to stop smoking as well as mothers. It will be very much easier for the mother to stop if she has the support and encouragement of the father, and if the father continues to smoke and leaves cigarettes lying around the house she is more likely to succumb to temptation. Two people attempting to stop smoking together are more likely to succeed than one person on their own, because one can help the other in moments of weakness.

You should also remember that smoking can reduce fertility in men, making conception less likely, and that there is also the problem for the mother of so-called 'passive' smoking, i.e. breathing in smoke put into the atmosphere by someone else in the family, which is also quite dangerous to non-smokers. After the baby is born it can also suffer from 'passive' smoking, and is very vulnerable at such a young age to this sort of pollution in the atmosphere. For this reason you should both continue to abstain from smoking after the baby is born. If a mother breastfeeds and starts smoking again she continues to put her baby at risk from yet another angle. All in all it is just not worth the risks, so both parents should make a concerted effort to give up smoking once and for all.

If you view life-long abstention with absolute distaste, resolve to stop just during pregnancy and while breastfeeding continues, and there is a good chance that in the meantime you will kill the habit for ever. Many women find that when they become pregnant they automatically lose their enthusiasm for smoking, as it can make morning sickness more severe. If this happens to you, use it to your advantage as a method to help you control your smoking habits, and eventually you may be able to stop smoking altogether. If you really cannot give it up completely, do still try to cut down as much as you can, as every little helps. Use anything you think might help – there are lots of anti-smoking aids on the market. Try them all if need be, as some methods suit some people better than others. Try anything, and remember that as a result you will also save money. In these days of economic gloom, the prospect of having extra money in the family might be the strongest incentive of all to stop smoking, especially when you are soon likely to have a potentially expensive baby on the way.

Alcohol

Until recently it was thought that drinking small amounts of alcohol occasionally just before or during a pregnancy was completely safe and would be unlikely to affect the baby in any adverse way. But several surveys have now been completed which show some alarming results, implying that even the occasional glass of wine or beer during early pregnancy, when the foetus is still developing, can be dangerous and can cause birth defects. Results of several surveys show that, among mothers who drank no alcohol at all during their pregnancies, significantly fewer babies had birth defects than among their counterpart mothers who drank moderately or 'socially'. Because of this I think that every mother-to-be should make a real effort to give up alcohol completely, if only for her own peace of mind. In fact many women find that they just can't tolerate any alcohol at all during pregnancy, because it often makes the symptoms of morning sickness and heartburn worse.

Excessive alcohol is always dangerous, so make sure you avoid real drunkenness if you are planning a baby, even before conception. You would be wise to do your best not to drink at all during the few months preceding a planned pregnancy, in order to avoid having drunk alcohol in the first few vital days after conception, when you may not realize that you are pregnant. The foetus is most vulnerable during the first three months of its life, and the first twenty-eight days are particularly dangerous if alcohol is taken, since this is when the first, crucial developments of the foetal nervous system take place. Really excessive drinking in the first few weeks of pregnancy can cause physical abnormalities and generally stunted growth, and if heavy drinking were to continue throughout the rest of the pregnancy the baby could be born mentally deficient too. In extreme cases you could lose your baby altogether. If you are taking any drugs, don't forget that they can affect the way in which alcohol works on you and may have some unpleasant side effects. Some drugs increase the effect of too much alcohol. If your doctor prescribes anti-sickness drugs for you in pregnancy, you should especially avoid drinking at the same time. There is no doubt that heavy drinking in pregnancy is inadvisable, and it now looks as if even social drinking may be potentially dangerous to your baby too, so, ideally, cut out all alcohol well before you conceive.

Drugs

It is difficult to avoid taking any drugs at all in our society, since so many are available over the counter in chemists' shops. Some drugs do not cross the placenta and are therefore safe for a prospective mother to take, but most of them do cross the placenta and enter into the baby's system. If you are contemplating pregnancy, cut out drugs completely, except those prescribed by your doctor. If, while you are preparing yourself for pregnancy, you need treatment from your doctor for any illness, tell him straight away that you are thinking about having a baby. In these circumstances he may prescribe a different drug, or he may ask you to take adequate precautions to prevent pregnancy until you have finished your course of treatment.

Remember that such apparently innocent things as aspirin or the caffeine in your coffee are also drugs, and that even these have an effect on the baby in your womb. Try to cut down on these or do without them both during pregnancy and in the months before conception. If in doubt, do without . . . remember that thalidomide was supposed to be safe. Any drug taken in excess is potentially dangerous, so if, for instance, you must take medicine to relieve a cough, keep to the dosage on the bottle. Better still, do without it altogether.

Illegal drugs such as marijuana, which many people use, are even more potentially dangerous since so little investigation has been made into their effects in pregnancy. Just because nobody has scientifically proved that marijuana is damaging during pregnancy doesn't mean that you can automatically assume it to be completely safe. Don't forget that as with all illegal practices you run the risk of prosecution if you use marijuana. The stress resulting from prosecution can be very upsetting and mentally unnerving at the best of times, let alone during pregnancy when your hormones often play havoc with your emotions. So refrain from illegal drug-taking completely while you are pregnant or while you are planning to conceive. All hard drugs, such as LSD, cocaine, amphetamines, heroin or morphine, should be avoided not only during pregnancy but also for six months before conception, so that there will be no risk of having taken any during those early weeks after conception when you may not realize you are pregnant. If you are addicted to any of these drugs, you should not consider becoming pregnant until you have first overcome the addiction and then spent at least six months without drugs in order to make sure that your body has returned to its normal state and that no traces of drugs are left in your system.

Tranquillizers and sleeping pills should also be avoided during pregnancy, if possible. If you are in doubt about any other drugs not mentioned here, ask your doctor's advice and listen to what he says.

The contraceptive pill

This needs a special mention because it is taken only by women of childbearing age and is therefore likely to be used during the months preceding a planned pregnancy. The one big problem with all the different varieties of contraceptive pill is that they can temporarily reduce fertility in some women. Quite a few women find that when they stop taking the pill after several years of using it they are unable to conceive straight away, and may have to wait for several months before becoming pregnant. This is probably because it takes a little while for the body to return to its normal cycle of menstruation. Since the pill can have this sort of effect on us after we have stopped taking it, it seems possible that it could also affect a growing foetus in some way. It must be pointed out that this is only a possibility – no one really knows for sure – but just to be on the safe side doctors are now recommending that women who stop taking the pill in order to conceive should actively prevent conception by some other means for 3–6 months to allow their bodies and menstrual cycles to return to normal. The most highly recommended alternatives are the barrier methods, i.e. the sheath or the cap. Since they are mechanical methods of contraception, they will not disturb the rhythms and cycles of your body and will allow your periods to return to their normal timetable, therefore ensuring that there is no residue of hormones left in your system which could in any way affect a growing foetus soon after conception. (The IUD is not recommended as a temporary contraceptive measure, since it directly affects the environment of the womb.) If you use this method of allowing your periods to become regular again before you conceive, you will also be able to work out your expected date of delivery more accurately when you do succeed in becoming pregnant.

Long-term medical problems

These include disorders like diabetes, epilepsy, continual high blood pressure and coeliac disease. If you suffer from any of these, or have any other long-term problem with your health, make sure you inform your doctor well in advance of your intention to conceive. There is no reason why any woman who suffers from this type of disorder should not happily rear a healthy family, providing the correct medical attention is given. There may be positive steps the doctor can take, and advice he can give you which could be very helpful for you to know in advance. If you have already been success-fully controlling a health disorder for any length of time and the condition is stable there is no reason why you shouldn't have a problem-free pregnancy; it is, however, important for your doctor to keep a careful check on your development and general health, and perhaps to look out for certain warning signs, so that if you do encounter any problems he will be able to take action early, before they have a chance to get out of hand. A prospective father who suffers from any long-term disorder should also talk to a doctor and tell him of his plan for fatherhood. Some disorders can be inherited, and if you or your future children are likely to be at risk in any way it is far better to know about it so that you can act accordingly and make balanced, well-informed decisions.

Sexually transmitted diseases

Before you attempt to conceive a baby it is advisable to make sure you are not suffering from any other medical conditions which need treatment. There are a whole range of sexually transmitted diseases that can affect a developing baby, and most people will know from their obvious symptoms if they are suffering from such a disease and will seek treatment. However, if you are in any doubt at all about whether you have such a disease when you decide to become pregnant, go and see your doctor straight away and have some tests to find out. If you have a vaginal discharge that doesn't seem quite right in some way or is different from normal, visit your doctor and ask his advice. If you suspect that your husband or partner is suffering from such a disease, encourage him to seek advice too. If either of you find you are infected in any way, it is important for *both* of you to undergo treatment before you consider pregnancy. Herpes, which is treatable but not curable, can cause complications in pregnancy if it is not monitored properly, but there need be no major problems so long as you take care to conceive in between attacks and have a high standard of hygiene. A herpes sufferer may be advised to have her baby delivered by Caesarian section, so as to avoid any infection being passed on via the vagina to the baby during birth. Whatever your medical problems there is usually a solution, so do consult your doctor well in advance of the possibility of conception and any risks can then be minimized.

German measles

German measles, or rubella, is only a mild illness in itself, but if caught by a woman in early pregnancy it can cause defects in the foetus, particularly hearing defects and problems with sight. If you know for sure that you had German measles as a child then you need not worry, as you will be immune to a further attack. If you are not sure or can't remember, you can ask your doctor to find out by looking up your medical history on your N.H.S. medical cards. If there is no indication that you either had the disease or were protected against it by an immunization injection, you should take great care to avoid coming into contact with it during the first few months of your pregnancy. If you are already pregnant you should try to ensure that you don't mix with anyone suffering from this illness. If you are still trying to conceive you can volunteer for the immunization injection, but this means that you will have to wait another few months before continuing to try to conceive, and you must be absolutely certain that you are not pregnant before going ahead with the injection. If you have any doubts or worries about German measles, consult your doctor.

Pollution

In our modern society we are constantly bombarded with pollution from every angle. When considering pregnancy it is important to try to minimize the amount of pollution confronting you before you conceive, so that your body is as free from chemicals as possible. You can minimize the effects of unavoidable pollution to a certain extent by eating the right kinds of nutritious foods, which will help to protect your system from the adverse effects of pollution in the environment. Eating a healthy diet over a long period of time means that your body will be in the peak of condition and ready and able to fight off infection, and will also help to counteract the effects of our polluted atmosphere. Good food safeguards you and your baby against the deleterious effects of pollution which cannot be avoided, such as smoke and industrial waste in the air, high levels of lead in the atmosphere surrounding main roads and motorways, and additives to the local water supply.

It is also a good idea to look at the conditions you work in. All modern factories where dangerous chemicals are used are subject to strict, rigorous health regulations and are checked periodically to see they adhere to the rules. However, if you work in a building where chemicals are used constantly in an industrial manufacturing process, it's worth checking up with a trade union health adviser or the local authorities to see if it is still safe for you to work there if you become pregnant. Fathers-to-be should also consider their places of work to make sure they are not being exposed to dangerous chemicals, since sperm can be adversely affected just as easily as an ovum or a growing foetus. Some chemicals, while not being dangerous to the foetus itself, can have the effect of reducing fertility in both men and women.

Hereditary diseases

These are diseases which are passed on from one generation to the next via the parental genes. Couples where one or both partners are suffering from a hereditary disease can often get specialist preconception advice from doctors who concentrate on the care and management of such diseases and who are particularly concerned with genetic counselling. The advice they give depends on each individual case, so if you think you need to see a genetic counsellor ask your own doctor to refer you to a specialist. Epilepsy and diabetes can be hereditary, but are not necessarily so, and the majority of people suffering from these two illnesses do not pass on the problem to their offspring. Hare lip, cleft palate, club foot, haemophilia, sickle cell disease, Down's syndrome and hydrocephaly are all hereditary. If you have previously had a baby suffering from one of these complaints, a genetic counsellor will be able to tell you the likelihood of your conceiving another affected child – this may not be as high as you fear, so it's worth finding out.

Weight

Your weight is an important factor to take into consideration before you conceive. Gaining weight in pregnancy is dealt with in greater detail in Chapter 1, but you should also think about your weight before you become pregnant at all. Look at Fig. 6 on p. 13. This shows approximate desirable weights for women before conceiving, in relation to their height and frame size. If your weight corresponds with that given in the chart for your height and frame size you need not worry, as a few pounds either way is not going to make very much difference. If, however, your weight is vastly different from that stated in the chart, you should consider doing something about it now, before you conceive. If you are seriously underweight you can make an effort to eat plenty of extra protein foods for a while, until your weight starts to increase, following the guidelines for a generally better-balanced diet given in Chapter 4. If on the other hand you are seriously overweight, now is the time to try to lose the excess baggage, before you conceive your baby. Give yourself plenty of time, limit your calorie intake to 1,000 calories per day, and try to keep the broad outline of your diet as well balanced as you can, eating plenty of fresh vegetables and fruit, a little protein, and cutting down on (but not cutting out) carbohydrates and fats. If you find difficulty in keeping to such a diet by yourself, you could try joining a slimming club for moral support. Some women find that while their previous efforts to slim have been unsuccessful, it becomes much easier when they have a real reason for slimming and a proper goal to aim for, such as a desire to conceive. When you reach your desirable weight, gradually increase your calorie intake again to maintain your weight at that healthy level. Give yourself another couple of months or so at this maintained, desirable weight before you try to conceive, as this will give your body a chance to stabilize before pregnancy starts adding on the pounds again. If you can follow the discipline of a calorie-controlled diet this will stand you in good stead for monitoring your weight gain throughout pregnancy itself, when you will be able to consume around 2,400 calories per day and, because you will have already mastered the sometimes elusive art of appetite control, will be less likely to 'let yourself go'.

Age

A woman's age is of primary concern when considering the optimum conditions for a first pregnancy, since with the aid of modern contraceptives we can now choose when we begin and extend our families. Gone are the days when teenage marriage automatically meant teenage motherhood, or when premarital sex ended more often in an unwanted pregnancy than in unmarried bliss. Now we can really choose when, or when not, to have a baby. Because of this, many women find that they want to balance career and children somehow, and often decide to dedicate their twenties and thirties to developing their job prospects so that they will have a career to return to after their babies are born. This sometimes results in a dilemma for such women, during their late twenties and early thirties, and they find they cannot decide what is the best age for them to have a baby. Many women worry that they should get a move on and have a first baby by the time they are thirty, while at the same time not wishing to forgo their hard-earned position at work just when they are at their working prime, when all that effort may be about to result in a step up on the work ladder, promotion to a higher position. Only the woman herself can weigh up the balance of these two things that she desires, and one may become more important to her than the other as time goes by, thereby resolving the problem. It is helpful, however, to know in more detail what problems the older mother faces to help her to make a well-informed and well-thought-out decision.

In fact there are two equally important points to consider

when establishing the ideal age to have a first baby: (1) physical prime, the best time to conceive from the body's point of view, and (2) emotional maturity, the ability to be able to cope with all the prospects and difficulties of childbirth and bringing up children. Ideally the mother-to-be will have had a chance to have seen something of the world, have faced and overcome a few problems, and be fairly realistic as to the responsibilities of pregnancy and motherhood, while at the same time still being in good shape physically. Statistics seem to prove that first-time mothers who are near the middle of their 'reproductive age' appear to have fewer complications, and give birth to fewer babies suffering from malformations and congenital abnormalities, than mothers who are very much older or very much younger.

A woman's age is also linked with fertility, as this starts to drop after the age of twenty-five. The deterioration is fairly slow to begin with, however, so that a woman of thirty still has a good chance of conceiving easily, while she may find it considerably more difficult at thirty-five.

To sum up, doctors seem to agree that while the majority of pregnancies at any age have a happy ending with a healthy baby and a healthy mother, there is a slightly greater risk of complications occurring in pregnancies which take place either near the beginning of a woman's fertile life, in the early teens, or at the end, from the age of thirty-five until after the menopause. However, don't worry, if you belong to one of these two age groups, as the risks of pregnancy in both groups can be minimized by good antenatal care. It cannot be stressed too much that the earlier in pregnancy you go to your doctor the better.

Sleep

An important part of preparing for pregnancy is making sure you get enough sleep. Sleep requirements vary from person to person, but most of us normally need around eight hours. It is important to rest well while you are trying to conceive, since you may find that during the first few months of pregnancy your sleep pattern is disturbed and you may suffer from insomnia. It is important that you are not tired out to begin with, as you will start your pregnancy at a disadvantage. To be in the peak of condition you need adequate sleep. Sleep works as a beauty treatment too – lack of sleep causes dark rings and bags around your eyes, and tired-looking skin, but if you get plenty of sleep these will disappear again and make your complexion and whole appearance very much better. So if you must have the odd late night on a special occasion while you are trying to conceive, try to make up for it the following day by sleeping late or having an early night. You should try to avoid taking sleeping pills at this time, as they can cross the placenta and may have some effect on a newly-formed foetus.

Stress

Stress is a hazard of our modern society, but you should try to avoid becoming too tense, stressed or upset while you are trying to conceive. Constant occurrences of this kind can sometimes cause real, physical illness, for example migraine headaches or skin irritations and rashes, and this is not conducive to a trouble-free pregnancy. Depression and anxiety can lead to serious health problems, so do try to sort out any worries and problems before you conceive. If you suspect that you may be suffering from a seriously depressive illness, you should seek help from a qualified doctor before attempting to conceive a baby – not because the baby's physical health itself will be directly affected by your depression, but because you may find it more difficult to cope with pregnancy and childbirth and possibly be more prone to long-term postnatal depression. Help *can* be given, so don't despair, but consult your doctor. Some mental disturbances can cause hormone levels to fluctuate, which could also affect your level of fertility for a while.

Don't go to your doctor asking for or expecting to get tranquillizers. These can cross the placenta and tranquillize the foetus as well as yourself, which may not be a good thing early on in pregnancy when the foetus is just starting to develop. If your doctor suggests tranquillizers without your prompting, make sure that he knows you are trying to conceive a baby – some tranquillizers are more suitable and safer for pregnancy than others. Remember that tension of any sort is not good prior to conception or during pregnancy. Relaxation is the name of the game when you are preparing yourself to carry a baby, so take up a relaxing pastime such as yoga, or make an effort to sit down in a comfortable chair with a good book and put your feet up for an hour or so every evening. If you feel yourself tensing up during the day, take a long, hot, relaxing bath in the evening and try to consciously unwind and let your mind wander where it will.

Exercise

The amount of exercise you normally get before you become pregnant depends largely on your lifestyle. If you drive to and from work every day and sit at a desk all day long, and if watching television or reading are your favourite pastimes, then you're not likely to use your muscles very much at all. If, however, you walk or cycle to work, have the sort of job that involves moving about, for example traffic warden, and have pastimes such as swimming or tennis, you'll be doing fairly well for exercise and should be quite fit as a result. Unfortunately not many of us have this kind of lifestyle, and it is probably true to say that most of us don't get as much exercise as we should – but why is it necessary to exercise at all, and what are the benefits of exercise for a woman planning a pregnancy in the near future? The answers are quite simple. If you want to be really fit and healthy when you conceive, you will need to be physically in good shape. You can eat all the right foods, give up smoking and other bad habits, be the right weight for your height, and generally do yourself an awful lot of good, but if your body isn't 'fit' as well you could still be neglecting one important facet of good health for pregnancy. This *doesn't* mean, however, that you need to struggle out into the midday heat for a ten-mile run every day, or exert yourself in any extreme way – this is more likely to be harmful than helpful. Instead it means that you will derive great benefit from just a few minutes every day of some regular, reasonably active, animated movement which will build up your strength and stamina gradually. A little effort every day is far more valuable than an exhausting workout once a week.

What is fitness

For your body to be really fit, several factors must be taken into consideration. First there is the need to make sure that your muscles and joints work properly and are in good condition. Muscles benefit from being used: unlike machinery which wears out through use, muscles are rather like living elastic and get stronger the more you stretch them. During and before pregnancy, there are special exercises you can do to use the muscles which are used in birth and delivery (see pp. 174–5). This involves knowing not only what and where these muscles are, and how to tense them and exercise them, but also how to relax them. Secondly there is the question of stamina and strength. Stamina is acquired through *regular* gentle or moderate exercise. Just a few minutes each day on a regular basis will soon build up your strength and your ability to carry on beyond your normal exhaustion threshold. You will need stamina during pregnancy, and especially during labour. Giving birth is a strenuous occupation – you will need all the stamina you can muster so that you will not only get through it comfortably, but will also enjoy it. Thirdly, the internal muscles of your body, such as the heart and the muscles surrounding the lungs, also need exercise. This is usually accomplished automatically when you take any exercise, because physical exertion makes the heart beat faster, thus exercising the heart muscle and making it stronger and capable of taking extra stress.

It must be emphasized that while you are trying to conceive you should not suddenly lurch into great physical activity if you have not been used to it before. Please remember the two most important words in this section – *gradual* and *regular*. Any physical movement will do if it makes your heart beat just a little bit faster, for example cycling, tennis, lively walking, keep-fit exercises, swimming or disco dancing. Some women get all the exercise they need from dancing to their favourite music at a disco or club. (This is admirable provided they don't spoil the effect by downing half a bottle of gin at the same time.) It is important to remember that whatever exercise you choose, you should build up a gradual routine that leaves you feeling refreshed and re-energized. You should not end up in a pathetic heap on the floor, too exhausted to move a single muscle afterwards (if this happens to you then you are straining too hard, so slow down and do it more gradually, building up your strength as you go).

Once you become pregnant there are some particularly strenuous activities which you should not continue to do, such as horse riding and skiing, but generally speaking, most gentle exercise is safe and beneficial during pregnancy. You may not be able to keep up your former track record of activity as your pregnancy progresses, but if you keep up just a small portion of it, even if it's just taking the dog out for a walk each day, you will continue to benefit.

If you have previously suffered a miscarriage or threatened miscarriage, you should not take vigorous exercise but should be guided by your doctor's advice.

Fresh air

During pregnancy it is a good idea for lots of reasons to get out and about in the fresh air, and it is as well to get into the habit before you conceive. One of the reasons we need fresh air and sunshine is because Vitamin D is formed in the body by the action of sunlight on the skin. This vitamin is essential for mothers-to-be because it aids the absorption of calcium into the body, and calcium is needed in quantity by all growing babies in the womb to form their bones during early pregnancy. This is not the only source of Vitamin D, since it is also present in some foods, but it is a pleasant and useful way of supplementing the amount you take in.

Just as the body takes in fuel and nutrients in the form of food, it also needs a regular quantity of good quality oxygen too. When you breathe in air with your lungs you breathe in oxygen, which is one of the main constituents of air. From the lungs this oxygen is transported to the blood, which has the job of carrying it around your body, depositing some wherever your body cells need it. The cells of a growing baby in the womb need a good supply of fresh, clean oxygen too, and this is transported to the baby from your bloodstream via the placenta. While it is true that you can't avoid breathing and therefore cannot suffer from a deficiency of oxygen, you should also consider the quality of the air you breathe. Those of you living in large, smoky cities would do well to make an effort to visit the country occasionally, to get the benefit of some really clean, pure, pollution-free air in your lungs. If you work in an office where other people smoke all day and the windows are kept shut you will be breathing in stale, smoky air all day long, so it is worth making the effort to keep a window near you open slightly, or to make sure you get outside and breathe some fresh air once in a while.

Pregnancy can also cause sleepless nights, and plenty of fresh air will help to counteract this. A brisk walk in the country or in a park always leaves me nicely tired out without exhausting me completely – just the state you should aim for.

4

Preconception Diet

Although this chapter is about diet before conception, its guidelines should also be followed during pregnancy itself. After pregnancy, in fact, it will provide a continuingly healthy diet for all the family. It includes a wide range of ideas for improving your nutrition, to help you change your old unhealthy food habits into a much more carefully thought out, planned, healthy regime. This is obviously particularly useful for a woman to follow before pregnancy, so that her body can prepare itself to receive and nourish a growing foetus, but it can also be used by a prospective father, since it is just as important to produce a healthy sperm as it is to produce a healthy egg. During pregnancy itself the diet can be continued, especially during the first twelve weeks of pregnancy when the foetus is initially forming. Ideally, the basic rules of good eating will continue after the baby is born. Your new baby can be encouraged from the start to recognize wholesome ingredients and reject the less nutritious fare, acquiring good eating habits from the cradle.

The need to eat well before you conceive

For maximum preconceptual health, as we have already seen, it is important for both parents to do away with certain things in their lifestyle such as cigarettes, alcohol and drugs. But we must also consider what should be put *into* the body to make it perform at its best. The human body needs the right fuel to make it function correctly. This of course involves choosing the food you eat and the liquid you drink, and knowing which foods are good and nutritious and which are less desirable. In Chapter 2 we looked at nutrition before conception, and how your nutritional needs change during pregnancy. In this chapter we will be considering how to choose the best foods to fill those nutritional needs both before and during pregnancy. In fact, your diet need not change very greatly during pregnancy if you have got the groundwork right beforehand. If you eat the right sort of healthy food before you conceive, you will hopefully have trained yourself and your partner into good habits by the time the baby is actually on the way. During the last two-thirds of your pregnancy you will merely have to increase your intake by about 300 calories per day, while making sure that you spend this extra daily calorie allowance on the right kind of nutritious foods.

Your food is your foundation for life

This reflects that famous old saying, 'You are what you eat'. The food you eat is, through the process of digestion and absorption, turned into *you*, your flesh, your skin, your hair, your nails, your body. Eating healthy foods will benefit you visibly – you will look better on the outside as well as feeling better inside. The existing cells in our bodies are repaired and replaced by the nutrients from our food, and the quality and strength and health of those new cells depends on the quality of the food taken in. You can't renovate an old building successfully with broken, crumbly, second-class bricks – you need good, strong, flawless bricks to rebuild it best. When you change your old eating habits and replace junk foods with a healthy diet, there is a gradual, noticeable improvement in all aspects of your body. Your hair gains more lustre and shines, your nails stop splitting and become stronger and tougher, your skin becomes clearer and loses its muddy grey appearance, you may sleep better, feel better, have more energy, and you may even lose some excess poundage and slim down a little. Good health through good nutrition shows itself in a myriad of ways. Little by little you will notice the difference, as the old cells in your body wear out and are replaced with new, stronger ones. You will start noticing the difference yourself fairly soon, but after six months of following the preconception diet other people will notice it too. Slowly your body adjusts and responds to the better quality fuel you are supplying it with. Slowly but surely your body benefits from the care you take over feeding it properly. Soon you feel ready to take the next important step – your body is healthy and fit, ready to receive a growing foetus and nurture it in the womb to bring it to maturity for birth. Time and time again I have seen it happen, this blossoming of health and vitality through thoughtful diet and careful nutrition.

Good food need not be expensive. You don't have to spend pounds and pounds of your hard-earned money on faddy health foods in high-class grocers and wholefood shops. Their prices have to be high because they are small shops with a low turnover, but supermarkets and chain stores all over the country are responding to the demand for more natural, healthy, fresh, unadulterated foods and are supplying them at competitive prices at last. In any case, fresh, unadulterated foods are quite often much cheaper than their processed alternatives, since fresh food doesn't carry the added expense of processing, of adding preservatives and colourings, or of being presented in expensive five-colour printed cardboard packets. Often the cheapest foods available are fresh fruit and vegetables in season, and what better place to start to improve your diet than with the plentiful supply we have in this country.

Good food need not be boring either. Choosing good food is mostly common sense, and if you follow the guidelines in this chapter you will soon learn to recognize the telling signs that indicate the less nutritious fare. Once you know what to look for and what to avoid it's easy. After a short while it will become second nature to you to eat only healthy, body-building foods, and hopefully you will have trained yourself and your partner into good eating habits which will last you for the rest of your lives and will also prepare the way for your children's eating habits. They will follow suit right from the start, since they will be well fed and nourished not only as babies but also while they are still in the womb. And even before they were conceived, your joint efforts as parents towards preconception care and diet will have paved the way for their good health and survival.

Building a baby

Some people are surprised to discover that a foetus in the womb is already perfectly formed in shape and that all the major organs of its body are constructed and working by the time it is twelve weeks old. After the twelfth week there is not very much that can go wrong with the development of the baby's body itself, and the remainder of the pregnancy just gives the baby time to grow in size and maturity until it can survive independently outside the womb. This is why it is so important to eat wisely *before* and during the early, formative days of pregnancy, especially in the weeks before conception and up to the twelfth week afterwards. These first twelve weeks of life are the crucial time when the baby's body is formed, when the important internal organs are built, when the arms and legs are growing and pushing their way out into properly formed limbs, and this is the vital stage where things can go wrong if any poisonous substance or drug which might cause a malformation in the foetus is taken by the mother.

The baby's body is built up from the nutrients the mother eats. It is ironic that, during the most vital time of development for the baby, the mother herself may not actually even realize she is pregnant. Thus she may not be aware of the need to take extra care over her diet in order to supply the growing baby with the right building materials, and to keep away from potentially harmful substances that might affect the foetus's development. Now, at last, we are able to take action before conception takes place. In these days of clever and convenient contraception we can choose when we conceive much more easily, and having that choice we can prepare our bodies for the event, and be caring and responsible parents even before the baby exists. The tiny spark of life can then grow and thrive in near optimum conditions, existing as it does inside your own body, drawing on the reserves stored up by you beforehand in readiness for just such an occasion.

Storing up good things for the future

Some of the nutrients in the food we eat accumulate in our bodies as stores which can be drawn on later when needed for a specific purpose. This can be useful when preparing for conception. One such nutrient is iron, which is stored in the liver. Women, in particular, need a good store of iron because they lose some every month during the menstrual period. In pregnancy the need is even greater, because the mother's body needs to manufacture a greater volume of blood so that she can cope with the growing bulk and metabolism of the baby, and because the baby's blood itself has to be manufactured from the mother's store of nutrients. The baby also needs a good store of iron in its own liver, because after it is born its main food for several months will be milk, which does not contain very much iron. So the baby needs enough iron stored in its liver to last it for 4–6 months after its birth. With such a great demand for iron in pregnancy, it is obviously a good idea to start eating more iron-rich foods before you conceive, so that when you need it most, at the beginning of pregnancy, you will have a good reserve. If you like you can also take an iron supplement for a few months before you plan to conceive – if possible, find one that includes folic acid, because this is partly responsible for the making of new red blood cells, and while it is found in some foods, particularly green, leafy vegetables, it is easily destroyed by cooking.

Some vitamins are also stored in the body. Water-soluble vitamins are *not* stored in the body, so you need to get a daily dose of those from your food. However, fat-soluble vitamins *can* be stored in the body, and these include Vitamins A, D, E, and K. If you eat a well-balanced, varied diet you should get enough of these fat-soluble vitamins without taking extra supplements in the form of pills, because they are needed only in minute amounts. In fact, simply because they *can* be stored, you should take particular care not to overdo your intake of this type of vitamin, since any excess is not excreted and this means that there is a possibility of overdose and poisoning occurring.

Water-soluble vitamins, however, are different. These include the Vitamin B group, Vitamin C, nicotinic acid, biotin, pantothenic acid and folic acid. (See 'Water-soluble vitamins', pp. 40–42.) They can be taken in pill form in any quantity completely safely, since any excess will be excreted by the body. However, it must be emphasized that it is far cheaper and probably better for you to get all the vitamins and minerals you need from your diet, with the exception of iron and, possibly, folic acid, both of which are specifically useful and can be in short supply in women of childbearing age.

The spina bifida connection

Recent research* has shown that there is a connection between the incidence of spina bifida and a deficiency of vitamins. Nobody is quite sure which vitamin is involved, if indeed the condition is caused solely by the lack of any particular one. It is now thought that spina bifida and certain other birth malformations, collectively known as neural tube defects, are probably caused not by one single influence but by several or many. The correction of only one of these, for example diet, could be enough to tip the scales in favour of a healthy child instead of a crippled one, and one of these many possible causes seems most definitely to be linked to the absence of vitamins in the diet in early pregnancy and before conception takes place.

In experiments recently conducted in this country, vitamins were given before and during pregnancy to women who already had one child affected by neural tube defects (NTD). The incidence of NTD in the subsequent babies of these

* 'Neural tube defects: prevention by vitamin supplements' by R. W. Smithells, *Pediatrics*, Vol. 69, No. 4, April 1982.

women was significantly lower compared with those of other mothers who also already had one child affected by NTD and who were not given any extra vitamins before and after conceiving again.

It is obviously very important to make sure that *you*, the woman now reading this book, get an adequate supply of vitamins and minerals before becoming pregnant and during your early pregnancy. I believe it is much better all round to obtain these essential nutrients entirely from natural sources, from wholesome food, rather than to take them in the form of synthetic supplements. But if for any reason you can't be *sure* that your diet is adequate in this respect, perhaps because you don't know enough about nutrition, or because you live out of a freezer, or because you continue to eat only processed, denatured foods despite what has been said here, then it is essential that you take a vitamin supplement as well. It is better to be safe than sorry. If in doubt, take a supplement before you conceive but do keep to the dosage on the bottle.

What is a wholesome diet?

How do you know which foods are the best? How do you know which foods to avoid? How can you put the basic rules of good nutrition into practice in order to benefit from them? The transition from sitting on the sofa reading about such good intentions to actually putting the ideas into practice in your own kitchen is not such a difficult step as you might imagine. You can start in a small way, concentrating on the obviously processed and denatured products in your larder to begin with. It may be obvious to you that custard powder is a processed, refined, artificially coloured food. So when you have finished the tin in your cupboard, don't buy any more. Instead, replace custard in your diet with more natural alternatives. If you still want custard you can make it, using unbleached flour to thicken the milk, and honey or malt extract to sweeten. Add egg yolks if you want to make it yellow, but why should it be yellow anyway? Only because you are used to it being so brightly coloured artificially. Why not have white custard instead? Being yellow doesn't make it taste any better, after all, so why bother? In this way you can gradually replace the refined products in your kitchen with more natural, wholesome alternatives. You will soon get to prefer the better flavours and will automatically choose wholesome ingredients for your cooking. Before going into detail and looking at each category of food more closely to find out how to make the changes, here are a few guidelines and basic ideas to set you on the right road.

1. Make sure you eat as many different kinds of food as possible. Try to eat some protein foods, some carbohydrate foods and some fresh fruit and vegetables each day.
2. Try to steer away from any food which is obviously processed, and look out for natural alternatives. Eat food which is as natural and as whole as possible. For example, use wholewheat flour instead of refined white flour, or steak, pot-roast or any whole cut of beef instead of processed beef sausages or beefburgers.
3. If you are not sure whether a particular product is good or bad, check the label. This may seem obvious, but many people don't bother. If the label states that the product contains lots of preservatives, artificial colourings or flavourings, put it back on the shelf and find a more natural alternative. For example, you'll find the list of ingredients on a packet of soup very long indeed. It will be full of things like anti-oxidants, emulsifiers, hydrogenated fats, monosodium glutamate and hydrolysed protein, etc., etc. Ugh. Try making your own soup instead. Processed meat products, i.e. pork pies or commercially made pâtés, are usually full of the same sort of unnatural ingredients. Remember, you are what you eat – do you really want your intestines and digestive organs constantly preserved, coloured, flavoured and emulsified by such products?
4. Try to eat fruit and vegetables in a more natural state – not tinned, not frozen, but fresh. Try to cook your fresh vegetables more carefully. Don't boil them to a mush, but

simmer them gently for just a few minutes, or sauté them. Even better, eat them raw.

5. Look out for foods with more fibre, for example wholewheat flour and wholewheat bread. They are more filling and also aid your digestion. All types of pasta and other wheat products can be made from wholewheat grains instead of white, including products like semolina. Look out especially for wholewheat spaghetti and macaroni, which are becoming more and more popular and are now available in many supermarkets.

6. Don't fry so much of your food. Try baking it in the oven or heating it under a grill instead. For example, don't eat chips – have baked potatoes instead.

7. Use fresh dairy products. Don't use processed cheeses, but look out for real farmhouse cheese cut from the block. Fresh milk is better than dried milk powder. Avoid commercially made, highly sweetened yogurt – use 'live' yogurt or try making your own.

8. Track down invisible sugar in processed products. You don't actually *need* any sugar at all in your diet from a nutritional point of view, but it is often added to commercial products to make them more palatable. If you happen to fancy something sweet occasionally that's fine, but watch out: sugar is added to lots of foods where you might not expect to find it, for example tinned or frozen peas, baked beans, tinned soups, tinned sweetcorn, and even many processed meat products. You will be better off without sugar, except for an occasional treat. Remember, *read the label*.

9. Eat fewer obviously sugary things. Cut down on biscuits, cakes, ice creams, jellies, custards and sweets. Eat dried and fresh fruits and honey instead, or restrict yourself to an occasional treat.

10. Cut down on red meat and fatty meat products. Try to eliminate some of the animal fats in your diet and substitute vegetable fats and oils.

11. If your local supermarket does not stock the products you require, make a point of asking the manager why not and

request that he starts stocking them. A shop will stock anything that sells well. If there is enough demand for a certain type of product it will be included on the shelves for purely financial reasons, because it is good for business, regardless of any nutritional benefits it carries.

Meat, fish and poultry

Into this category come all the flesh foods that are obtained from animals, fish and birds, including offal. In these days of modern processing and mechanical, chemical preservation of foodstuffs, meat suffers rather badly – it is mashed, squeezed and pulverized, ground up and crushed, minced and shaped into many different forms. This in itself is not so *very* bad (I like nothing better than homemade liver pâté, which undergoes a similar mincing process), but the subsequent addition of so many artificial colourings, preservatives, emulsifiers, flavourings and other synthetic additives of various kinds turns what was once a nourishing piece of fresh meat into a nutritional graveyard. Meat which has been treated in this way by manufacturers in order to give it a shelf life of several months is unlikely to be very appetizing or nutritious, hence the added artificial flavours and colourings to bring it back up to 'standard' and make it taste better, and the artificially added vitamins to replace the natural ones destroyed by the processing. Personally, I would far rather have had that piece of meat in its original state and cooked it myself, before it was mutilated into a modern, denatured food product, and this is the view of most people who are concerned with making their diet more nutritious, natural and healthy.

REJECT: all manufactured, processed meat products, including commercially made sausages, pâtés, and meat pies; tinned ham, corned beef, tinned hot dog sausages, tinned meat balls; beefburgers, faggots, pork pies, ready-made shepherd's pies, etc., frozen savoury pancakes, fish fingers, fish cakes, battered fish, etc.

REPLACE WITH: whole joints of lean meat, for example beef, lamb or pork; chops, steaks, any fresh cuts of meat; bacon, real ham; fresh chicken, turkey, rabbit; homemade sausages, homemade pâtés and terrines; offal, for example liver and kidneys; freshly minced beef and pork; all types of fresh fish, shellfish, etc.

Meat

You may argue that fresh meat is much more expensive than the processed alternatives, but let's take a closer look. For instance, how much meat is there in a typical, processed pork pie? The proportion of meat is fairly low, so that you are actually paying a lot of money for the pastry that surrounds it and the jelly inside. If you can afford to buy the more expensive, lean cuts of meat, for example steak or joints of beef or lamb for roasting, all well and good. If not, there are many cheaper cuts available, for example chops, breast of lamb, oxtail, belly pork, best end of neck, spare ribs, stewing beef, offal, or cheaper cuts of bacon. These can all be used just as successfully and are just as nutritious as the more expensive cuts. Chops are versatile and can be baked, grilled or casseroled. Breast of lamb and spare ribs are good when baked at a high temperature to make them crisp and reduce the fat content, while breast of lamb can also be stuffed and rolled before baking. Best end of neck and stewing beef can be casseroled with different vegetables in season, and belly pork is good stewed slowly with beans and tomatoes. Liver and bacon are delicious baked in foil with an onion and some herbs. Try making your own liver pâté and meat pies, using minced meat. Kidneys are nice grilled for breakfast. When roasting whole joints of meat, don't forget to use up the juices that collect in the bottom of the pan – they are full of goodness. If you don't want to make gravy, just spoon off any excess fat and pour the remaining juices over your vegetables. Don't forget that you can buy meat bones from your butcher extremely cheaply, and they are good value for making soup. Any bones will do including cooked bones left over from roasts and raw bones such as oxtail, ribs, etc. Just simmer them gently with some vegetables. There is lots of goodness in the marrow from larger bones, and this gives soup a lovely flavour too. Use poultry carcasses in the same way. Some larger shops and supermarkets have their own butchery departments, and sometimes they sell misshapes of meat very cheaply. You may also be able to find misshapes of sliced bacon. Get to know on which days your local shop packages its meat and you'll know when to look out for these cheaper alternatives.

Fish

Buy fresh fish from a fishmonger or from your local market. Be adventurous – experiment with different types of fish that you may not have used before. Use fresh cod, coley, haddock, plaice, mackerel, trout, herring, skate, eel, halibut, turbot, whiting, whitebait, sole, bass, hake, mullet, salmon . . . the list is endless. Don't forget fish roes, they are very nutritious and there are many varieties cheaper than caviar to choose from. Include shellfish in your diet: cockles, mussels, oysters, scallops, whelks, winkles, crab, lobster, prawns and shrimps, for example. There are a few tinned fish, for example tuna, salmon, pilchards, and sardines, which are acceptable. These are relatively cheap and the tins contain only the fish itself and some oil or brine.

Smoked fish: Some work has been done recently on the incidence of diabetes in babies whose parents regularly ate chemically smoked food products before conceiving. (This includes products such as bacon and smoked meats as well as smoked fish). These tests were carried out in Iceland, where smoked food is often eaten in quite large quantities every day, and the evidence has yet to be conclusively proven. It is unlikely that an occasional meal containing a little smoked food will cause an imbalance in a foetus, but it is just as well to avoid *large* quantities of smoked products while preparing for conception until, and unless, the effects on the foetus have been conclusively proved to be harmless.

Poultry and game

This includes chicken, turkey, duck, goose, pheasant, grouse, rabbit, hare, pigeon, etc. Some of these may seem expensive to you, but you may be able to buy game more cheaply from friends who go shooting. I don't really like the idea of shooting game for pleasure, but if you know someone who does it anyway you might as well use the resulting rabbits, pheasants, etc. for food. Frozen chickens are better than ready-made commercial chicken products, but fresh chickens are better than frozen. Most frozen chickens are injected with chemicals to make the flesh retain more water, thereby making the flesh more 'juicy' and increasing the weight of the bird. Fresh chickens are almost bound to taste better, and be better value even if they do cost slightly more per pound, since some of the weight of a frozen bird may be due to extra water retained in the meat.

Eggs

There are many different kinds of eggs, although hen's eggs are usually the cheapest. Look out for duck eggs, often sparkling white or a lovely, soft green colour, or goose eggs which are enormous. You may find both of these in wholefood shops or on local produce market stalls, even in city centres. Different breeds of hens produce different types of eggs too – look out for the really dark brown, spotted ones laid by Black Marron hens, or see if you can find some bantam's eggs which are quite small. I always try to buy free range eggs, more out of consideration for the hens who have to lay them than for any nutritional reason.

Eggs are cheap and a very good supply of protein. They can be boiled, poached, scrambled, baked or made into an omelette. They can be incorporated into wholesome cakes or turned into delicious soufflés, they can be added to stuffings or put in sandwiches, they can be stirred into custard or whisked into milk shakes. In a word, eggs are *versatile*. They are excellent value for money, and just the job for mothers-to-be who need foods which are full of goodness without being full of calories too.

Dairy foods

These include milk and all milk products such as yogurt, all types of cheeses, butter, cream and buttermilk.

REJECT: skimmed milk, dried milk powder, long life milk, tins of condensed, sweetened milk; any processed cheeses, including commercial, processed cheese spreads; processed sweetened yogurt; cream substitutes, sweetened cream.

REPLACE WITH: whole, fresh cow's or goat's milk; real farmhouse cheeses cut from the round, natural soft cheeses such as Brie or Camembert, cottage cheese; 'live' un-sweetened yogurt; real cream, buttermilk; butter.

Whole, fresh milk is good protein for a growing baby in the womb and also provides valuable calcium. Commercial yogurt is packed full of sugar and chemical additives, so avoid it; look out for 'live' yogurt or make your own at home. Use yogurt instead of processed cheese spreads to make savoury dips, add it to soups, use it to top fruit salads, pour it over stuffed, savoury pancakes and use it as a low-calorie salad dressing. Real farmhouse cheeses taste better than plastic, processed cheese. If you want something akin to a cheese spread use a soft cheese like Brie, or make your own spread by making a very thick cheese sauce and letting it 'set' in the fridge to a spreadable consistency. Go easy on cream except as an occasional treat – it is very high in calories and contains mostly fat. Use buttermilk if you can find it (some supermarkets stock it regularly); add it to soups or whisk it up with some honey for a refreshing, cool drink. Use butter sparingly – it is best to limit its use to spreading on bread, where you can taste its richness. Use vegetable oils for general cooking, as they are cheaper and are not high in cholesterol like animal fats.

Oils and fats

This includes all solid fats and liquid oils produced from animal or vegetable sources.

REJECT: hydrogenated cooking fats (i.e. any artificially solidified fat made originally from a liquid oil); poor quality vegetable oils; commercial margarines, low calorie slimming margarines; lard, suet.

REPLACE WITH: unsaturated liquid vegetable oils such as sunflower, soya, safflower or sesame seed oils; butter (in moderation only).

Some people argue that lard and suet are natural products and should therefore be acceptable in a healthy diet. They are derived from animals and are therefore natural, it's true, but unfortunately they have a very high cholesterol content. Cholesterol in large quantities is not beneficial, especially to men, since it is connected with heart disease and with the high incidence of heart attacks in middle-aged and younger men. For this reason it is a good idea to cut down on animal fats in your diet and replace them with vegetable oils. You need not cut them out altogether, but do try to cut down. Try to do some of your cooking and baking using vegetable oils instead. For instance, it is quite possible to make good pastry with a liquid oil, using slightly less oil per weight of flour than you would if you used a solid fat. Thus for 12 oz of wholewheat flour you need only 4 fl oz of vegetable oil, plus a little salt to taste and enough cold water to mix. It saves all that 'rubbing in', too, as you can just mix the oil into the flour with a fork.

The best vegetable oils are those which are cold-pressed. This means that they have been extracted from the seeds, beans or kernels only by being mechanically crushed and then put under pressure from heavy weights, and have not been subjected to heat or chemicals to extract the oil. After all the oil that can be extracted by cold-pressing has been obtained, manufacturers of cooking oils resort to other methods to extract yet more oil from the plants or seeds.

This involves using heat and/or chemicals, and the oil that results from using these methods is always of a poorer grade than the cold-pressed variety. Cold-pressed oils are usually a bit more expensive, but they also taste better as they tend to retain the natural flavour of the plant or seeds from which they were extracted. Look out for good quality almond, soya, corn, olive and peanut oil.

Cereals and grains

Under this heading come all the different grains – wheat, barley, rye, millet, oats, corn, rice – and any product made from grains and cereals such as bread, pastry, etc.

REJECT: all processed wheat products, including white flour, white bread, white pastry, and white pasta; all processed baking products such as ready-made cake or pudding mixes; gravy mixes; custard powder; frozen white pastry; all commercial breakfast cereals; white rice.

REPLACE WITH: wholewheat products wherever possible, including wholewheat flour, wholewheat bread, wholewheat pastry, and wholewheat pasta; homemade cakes, biscuits and puddings, made with wholewheat flour; muesli or porridge; brown rice; any whole grain product.

It is only since the turn of the century that white flour and commercial white bakery products have become so popular. We now know that white, refined flour is not as good for us as wholewheat flour, because so much of the goodness is literally milled out of it – vitamins, minerals, roughage, etc. Modern, metal, high-speed roller mills cause the flour to singe and colour, so that it has to be chemically bleached white again before it can be sold. Stone ground flour is milled very slowly in comparison, and so does not need adulterating afterwards with chemicals. It is also now widely recognized that we need fibre in our food, and the fibre in wheat, which consists of the bran and wheatgerm, are taken out of white flour. Fibre is important because it is needed for good digestion, helping the food on its way through the bowel and preventing constipation. It is also very filling and can prevent us from over-eating, which is very important in pregnancy when the appetite may increase. So use only wholewheat products if possible. If you find you don't like the flavour or the texture to start with, use half wholewheat and half white for a while until you become used to it. Eventually you will come to prefer the better flavours and textures of natural food, and will not crave after the unhealthy sort of food you once ate.

As well as using wholewheat bread and flour, look out for wholewheat pasta. Wholewheat macaroni, spaghetti, noodles, lasagne, pasta rings, etc. are all available in wholefood stores and in some supermarkets. Make your pastry with wholewheat flour, and try adding some barley or rye flour to your baking occasionally. Use extra bran and wheatgerm in your cooking too, adding them to soups and stews and incorporating them into cakes and biscuits.

Commercial breakfast cereals are sprayed with synthetic vitamins because the manufacturing process is so damaging to the cereal. It is far better to eat grains and cereals which are in their natural state, with their natural vitamins and minerals still intact. Use muesli or porridge for breakfast, and make your own muesli in preference to using the ready packaged sort, since commercial varieties often contain lots of sugar. Making your own muesli is much cheaper too.

Don't just restrict your intake of grains and cereals to wheat. Muesli contains flaked rye, barley and wheat. Try popping your own popcorn, it's very cheap and it's fun too. No need to cover it with sugar, though: try sprinkling a little salt on it instead or eat it plain. Use brown rice instead of white – it tastes far nicer, nutty and delicious. (Remember to allow a slightly longer cooking time.) If you have some cold, cooked brown rice left over, use it to make a brown rice salad; just add a few nuts, some raisins and some sweetcorn kernels and mix well. Look out for the more unusual grains, such as bulghur, buckwheat or millet. Bulghur is wheat that has been chopped and roasted. Just soak it in cold water until soft, then strain and serve like rice, or simmer it gently until cooked if you prefer it hot. Buckwheat is not, strictly speaking, a grain, it's a seed, but it cooks like a grain and is good simmered gently for a few minutes with a little salt added. Millet also has an attractive nutty flavour, but make sure you cook it well, as it takes quite a lot of simmering to make it soft. Use whole grains of barley, wheat or oats in soup, along with a few lentils.

Dried beans, nuts and seeds

This includes all dried beans, peas and lentils, all types of nuts, and certain seeds such as sunflower, sesame and pumpkin seeds.

REJECT: processed bean products such as TVP (textured vegetable protein, obtained from soya beans); chocolate-covered nuts, sugared almonds, etc.

REPLACE WITH: whole dried beans, including soya, red kidney, blackeye, mung, haricot, aduki and butter beans, chickpeas, split peas, and lentils; nuts, shelled or unshelled, including almonds, walnuts, brazils, peanuts, cashews, pistachios, coconut, chestnuts; seeds, including sunflower, sesame and pumpkin seeds; peanut butter.

There are many different dried beans and peas available and they are a good source of cheap protein. You can use them as a substitute for meat, for example beans on toast, or bean burgers, or in addition to meat in dishes such as casseroled pork and beans, or chilli con carne. Chickpeas, cooked and mashed together with some lemon juice and garlic, make a very nice savoury dip. Mung beans can be sprouted for extra goodness, as this considerably increases the level of vitamins. Split peas and lentils make excellent soup. Nuts and seeds are good protein too: grind them up to add to nut roasts and other vegetarian dishes, add them to muesli or porridge, or make cakes and biscuits with them. Use nuts as a nutritious snack when you get that empty feeling between meals, instead of resorting to crisps or sweets.

Fruit

This includes all types of fresh and dried fruit.

REJECT: fruit tinned in heavy syrup; crystallized fruits; fruit frozen with sugar; tinned fruit pie fillings, commercial fruit pies, etc.

REPLACE WITH: all types of fresh fruit, including apples, peaches, apricots, bananas, oranges, lemons, grapefruit, plums, damsons, cherries, strawberries, raspberries, blackberries, gooseberries, blackcurrants, redcurrants, grapes, melon, pineapple, rhubarb, fresh dates and figs; all types of dried fruit, including raisins, currants, sultanas, apricots, prunes, figs, dried dates, pears, peaches, bananas and apples; fruit tinned in water or unsweetened fruit juice.

Fresh fruit is the best kind of fruit to eat – and it's so easy to chop up a few pieces of fresh fruit and mix them together to make an attractive fruit salad. Remember to leave on the skins of apples and pears. Fruit pies and puddings can be made with fruit purée: just simmer the fruit gently, with a little honey if you want to sweeten it, until it is soft and mashes to a purée with a fork. Look out for fruit tinned in water or unsweetened fruit juice; you may find it on the diabetic counter in a chemist's shop if you can't track it down in a supermarket. Mixed dried fruit makes a good snack or treat, especially dried dates, which are particularly sweet. Try some of the more unusual dried fruits, for example bananas, for a change.

Vegetables

REJECT: tinned vegetables, especially those which have added sugar, for example peas, sweetcorn, baked beans, etc. (restrict use of these if you cannot eliminate them altogether); frozen vegetables (use them occasionally for convenience but not on a regular basis).

REPLACE WITH: a good variety of fresh vegetables in season. *Green, leafy vegetables* include cabbage, Brussels sprouts, broccoli and calabrese, mustard and cress, lettuce, water-

cress, spinach, spring greens, curly kale, parsley and chives.
Root vegetables and tubers include carrots, parsnips,
swedes, turnips, beetroot, radishes, sweet potato, artichokes
and potatoes. *Fruit and seed vegetables* include cucumbers,
marrows, tomatoes, beans, peas, mushrooms, sweetcorn,
green or red peppers, aubergines, okra, courgettes, cauliflower, avocados, beansprouts, and olives. *Bulb vegetables*
include onions, shallots, spring onions, garlic and leeks.
Stem stalk and leafy stalk vegetables include celery, aspar-
agus, chinese leaf and chicory.

As you see, there are a great many vegetables available, and it
is a good idea to eat as many different kinds as you can. Buy
them as fresh as possible, and don't keep them in the fridge
for days before you cook them or they will lose much of their
goodness. Cook all vegetables as little as possible, or even
better, don't cook them at all – most vegetables can be eaten
raw in salads. Take special care when you cook green, leafy
vegetables, as the goodness in them is very easily destroyed
by overcooking. Cook them just long enough to heat them
through, don't boil them to a mush – they should still be
crisp. Greens are really best steamed, and it is well worth
investing in a steamer because so much goodness from
cooked vegetables is thrown out with the water they were
boiled in. Steamed vegetables taste better too, and keep their
colour and shape. Don't soak them in cold water before
cooking, as it has a similar effect to overcooking. If you must
boil your vegetables, make sure you keep the cooking water
to make soup. Leave the skins on root vegetables like potatoes and carrots, because much of the goodness of root
vegetables is found just under the skin, but make sure you
scrub them well first (a pan scourer makes a very good
vegetable scrubber).

Sugar

Sugar, whether white, granulated sugar or dark brown mus-
covado, is not actually needed in the diet at all. It is not an

essential nutrient needed by the body in order to carry out any special function, in the way that protein or vitamins are, for example. Of course the body needs simple 'sugars' such as glucose to function properly, but in fact all the glucose the body needs is manufactured independently inside the digestive system, from carbohydrates or from excess protein, so that the sort of crystallized white sugar I am referring to here is really surplus to requirements in our diet. In fact, sugar is totally undesirable, because of the adverse effects too much of it can have on our bodies – it makes us fat, rots our teeth, and is in its own way addictive, leading us into the bad habit of craving further sweet-tasting things to eat. The calories in sugar (112 per oz) are all 'empty' calories, which means they serve only to be turned into fat and stored in our bodies, and have no useful, nutritional function at all. In short, this means that we could all benefit greatly by cutting sugar out of our diet completely. This is certainly worth aiming for, although difficult to achieve, I admit. So as far as sugar and your health goes, *aim* at eventually cutting it out of your diet altogether. In the meantime, eat sugary things just occasionally – when you particularly fancy something sweet, or when it's your birthday, or when you're celebrating a special event.

Part of the problem in cutting down on sugar in your diet is actually establishing where it is to be found in your food. If you eat only natural foods you will know when you are eating sugar, because you will be cooking your own meals and will know what goes into them. If, on the other hand, you eat a large amount of processed convenience foods, you may be surprised to find that many of them contain a high proportion of sugar. Even meat products and other savoury products you might not normally suspect can be full of invisible sugar, so watch out for it by checking the list of ingredients on the label, as well as cutting down on the obviously sugary items. It will take time for your body to adjust to your new diet, so do it gradually, so that it will not be a noticeable shock to your system. This way you won't start craving sweet things to fill the gap.

REJECT: all sugary, processed bakery products, including instant cake mixes, commercial cakes and packets of biscuits; sugary jellies, jams, ice creams, all confectionery, custard, icings, puddings, sugar-coated breakfast cereals; sugary tea and coffee; chocolate; fruit tinned in heavy syrup; fizzy, sweetened drinks, sweetened fruit squashes; tinned peas, sweetcorn and baked beans; tomato ketchup (yes! look at the label); some tinned soups, etc., etc. The list is almost endless. If you must eat any commercial, processed junk food do remember to read the label, and if sugar is on the list, put it back on the shelf.

REPLACE WITH: naturally sweet foods such as dried fruits, fresh fruit and honey; malt extract, maple syrup, molasses and fruit purées. Make your own cakes and biscuits, and try to use honey or dried fruit to sweeten them, for example date slice or almond flan, which don't really need sugar.

There are many ways in which you can make sweet treats for yourself without using any sugar. Sweeten fruit with honey, sweeten homemade custard with malt extract, make milk shakes with honey or maple syrup. Rich fruit cakes can easily be made without sugar – just follow your usual recipe but leave the sugar out. You'll find that this won't make much difference to the texture or the flavour, and it will still be very sweet because of all the dried fruit. Make your own jelly by dissolving honey in fruit juice and setting it with gelatine. Make milk jellies in a similar way. Make your own ice cream by whipping together some cream, soft fruit and honey, and putting in the freezer. If you really must have something sugary now and then for a treat, make it yourself, so that even if you're hooked on the sugar you can at least avoid the chemicals and preservatives.

Drinks

What you drink is just as important as what you eat. There are a lot of adulterated drinks in our shops and supermarkets as well as adulterated foods, so take care over choosing the liquids you consume.

REJECT: fizzy 'cola'-type drinks, pop, lemonade, orangeade, etc. – these are all loaded with sugar and also contain many artificial preservatives and colourings. The same goes for commercial fruit squashes, lemon barley water, or sugary blackcurrant cordials. Avoid instant coffee, sweetened hot chocolate drinks, commercial milk shake mixtures, and alcohol.

REPLACE WITH: real unsweetened fruit juice from a carton or bottle, for example orange, pineapple, apple or grapefruit juice; tomato juice, other vegetable juices; unsweetened tea or coffee, iced tea and coffee (use real percolated coffee and drink it only occasionally, as it is a strong stimulant); milk, plain water from the tap, bottled mineral water; egg nog, hot yeast extract drinks.

Try whisking or liquidizing yogurt and soft fruits together and drinking through a straw. Or use buttermilk as a base for cool, refreshing drinks. Add a beaten egg to milk shakes – it adds 'froth' and makes it very bubbly when whisked, as well as making it more nutritious.

Note: As usual, reading about a good idea is easier than actually putting it into practice. The spirit may be willing but the flesh is more likely to be weak. The ideas in this chapter represent an ideal situation, a near perfect diet, which is something to be aspired to though not necessarily accomplished completely by everyone. I know only too well what a slow process changing your diet can be, but don't make this an excuse to go on mindlessly eating junk foods when you know they are not good for you.

Do, however, make a real effort to follow these dietary guidelines just a little when you are pregnant or preparing yourself for pregnancy, for the sake of your own health and that of the baby you carry, or will carry, inside your womb. Remember that this child depends on you for its continued existence, and for all the nourishment it needs to grow into a viable human being. Try your best to do it justice, to help it develop to its full potential, and to provide it with the best raw materials you can possibly give it, to enable it to grow healthily and give it a good start in life. Once you have got yourself and your family into good eating habits, you will have established a good dietary basis which will serve you for the rest of your life and which will also encourage your children along the right lines from the beginning.

5

Looking Good in Pregnancy

Looking good

When you are pregnant you can either feel marvellous, look on top of the world and appear radiant and blooming for twenty-four hours every day, or you can feel absolutely lousy all the time, wanting to crawl off into a dark corner somewhere and feeling so miserable that you begin to wish you weren't pregnant at all. Many of us come somewhere between these two extremes for much of the time, but as our pregnancies progress, most of us suffer from an increasing conviction that we are fat, frumpy and unattractive. This is partly due to the fact that we are simply unaccustomed to our present size, and can therefore easily panic over our appearance. There are many complex reasons why pregnant women encounter these sweeping changes in their moods and emotions, ranging from changing hormone levels, the favourite reason given these days, to plain boredom and frustration at not being able to physically move around freely, and at the inevitable clumsiness of the last few weeks of pregnancy.

One of the best remedies for this depressed feeling is to take a little care over the way you look, and to spend some time grooming yourself. Try to remember that your condition is not permanent! Your baby *will* be born and you will regain your figure in due course. This lumpiness is only a temporary stage – it won't last for ever. Of course you may feel perfectly happy with your figure and wonderfully fulfilled, in which case you are one of the lucky ones. But if, like most of us, you have bleak moments of desperation over your enlarging apparatus and your diminishing attractiveness, don't just sit there wallowing, get up and do something about it.

Clothes

Clothes obviously play a big part in the way you feel about yourself. We all know what a refreshing feeling it can be to go out and buy some new clothes or dress up for a special occasion. (This is not a sexist view of women – men like dressing up too.) The clothes you wear make a statement about the type of person you are, they tell other people about your character, they reflect your lifestyle and state of mind, and this is just as true during pregnancy as at any other time. The problem with pregnancy is that unless from the very beginning you wear enormous tents that will take you right through the following nine months, you'll find that you grow out of everything remarkably quickly. Of course you can go out and buy new maternity clothes as you need them, but few of us can afford to buy as many as we would like. So what is to be done? Don't worry, there are lots of things you can do to stretch your existing wardrobe to accommodate your pregnant state. First of all, take a good look at the clothes you have. Go through everything, and sort out all the clothes that may still fit you during the first few months, before you get too large. Do you have any loose smock shirts or flowing dresses? You might come across an old caftan, or a skirt with an elasticated waist. You are almost certain to have some things that will keep you going for a while. Perhaps you possess a large, wrap-around coat or a cape? Baggy dungarees are fashionable and comfortable, and many sweatshirts are big and loose enough to give you some room for expansion. Large loose-knit jumpers will cover up and hide your growing lump very nicely. In this way you can lay the foundations of your maternity wardrobe.

Even though hopefully you won't be putting on too much weight to start with (around 10 lb during the first four or five months), you will probably find that even this will be enough to make many of your present clothes unserviceable. In early pregnancy, any tight-fitting clothes or constriction around your middle can have the unpleasant effect of increasing morning sickness and general nausea. Some women find right from the start that they can't bear any feeling of tightness at all around the middle, as it makes them feel sick. So any tight jeans, well-fitting trousers or skirts with waistbands which fit you perfectly now could soon disappear off your wearable list. Even though your weight may not increase much to begin with, you may find that your stomach and breasts swell enough to prevent you fitting into your present clothes. Other people probably won't notice any visible difference at this stage, but you could feel very uncomfortable if you don't start wearing some looser clothes.

It's worth asking around your friends and family to see if anyone has any maternity clothes you could borrow or buy second-hand. Most women who have recently become mothers are likely to be fairly sympathetic to the problems of dressing yourself during pregnancy, and will be only too glad to help. (Remember to do the same for any other pregnant friends after your own baby is born.) Don't forget to ask your mother and/or mother-in-law. (Yes, I know you wouldn't normally dream of wearing your mother's clothes but it's worth asking just in case, especially as mothers are generally a very good source of baggy nighties, something you'll need plenty of if you are opting to have your baby in hospital.) If your partner is at least one size bigger than you are normally, delve into his cupboards too (ask him first of course!). He's bound to have some big jumpers and loose-fitting shirts that will do very well. You may be able to wear jeans a bit longer too if you borrow his.

Perhaps you could make some clothes yourself. Not everyone is good at sewing and knitting, but those of you who are can take advantage of your skill now, particularly if this is your first baby and you are giving up work early. There are some fairly easy sewing patterns which anyone with even limited sewing experience can make up successfully. Most patterns for maternity clothes are loose and wide, so there is little fitting involved and no careful shaping to get right.

Many women find that they perspire more freely during pregnancy, and need clothes which let the air through and allow the skin to 'breathe'. Ideally they should be made of fairly absorbent material. Synthetic materials like nylon are not very good during pregnancy because they can make you so sweaty. Natural fibres are best – look out for 100 per cent cotton or linen fabrics, cotton mixtures (with a high percentage of cotton), or silk if you can afford it. Corduroy, needlecord, cotton velvet, denim and towelling are all cotton based. Choose woollen fabrics for heavier garments, and try to avoid acrylic and synthetic materials. Jumpers should be made from wool, or from yarn that has a high percentage of wool fibres (these will be warmer too). For your own sake try to buy clothes that are machine washable, as you won't feel much like standing at the sink washing clothes by hand when you are eight months pregnant. Try to wear fairly light-weight clothes that feel comfortable and are airy. It is a good idea to choose clothes that you are likely to wear after the birth too. Most maternity dresses can be tied with a belt and worn successfully afterwards. If you are planning to breastfeed, look out for tops and dresses that unbutton down the front to the waist – this makes breastfeeding easier.

You will need different maternity clothes according to what time of year your baby is due to be born. If you are likely to be at your largest during midsummer, you should manage quite easily by investing in a few floaty dresses. If you are likely to spend the end of your pregnancy during the winter months, however, you will need some warmer clothes as well, for example a large wrap-around coat, cape, shawl or poncho, and warm, woolly tights that are big enough to go around a forty-inch waist. If you find that your legs ache a lot and you tire easily as pregnancy progresses, you could try wearing support tights. If you don't want to wear tights at all, try leg-warmers or over-the-knee socks. To look their best, maternity smocks and dresses really need to be fitted around the shoulders and arms, as this allows them to hang properly without looking too bulky. Skirts can be elasticated at the waist or tied with a draw-string. Any trousers which have an elasticated waist or a draw-string will be comfortable and look good up to about the sixth or seventh month, or you can buy special maternity trousers – these have a large, elasticated front panel which will keep on stretching right up to delivery. Look out for boiler suits, dungarees and jumpsuits that are baggy enough to cover the bulge. If you don't want to buy special maternity clothes, go for ordinary clothes two sizes bigger than your usual size. Look in Indian boutiques, which usually have many gathered, fuller styles. Try your local 'nearly new' shop too – maternity clothes often turn up in second-hand shops when mothers have no one else to pass them on to. The choice is yours. Whatever you choose, enjoy the change, and just to record the event ask someone to take some photographs. After the baby is born you may not believe you were ever that big.

Underwear needs a special mention. There is no doubt that cotton underwear is best during pregnancy; it lets your skin breathe at a time when your sweat glands may be working overtime, and it is far more absorbent than other materials. You can buy special maternity knickers which have a stretchy panel, or you can wear ordinary bikini briefs which cover the essential parts but leave the bump uncovered. Deciding what to do about a bra is another matter. Many women these days don't wear a bra under normal circumstances but wonder whether they should do so in pregnancy. It is really just a matter of how comfortable you feel, and how large you are normally. I have never worn a bra during pregnancy or at any other time, except for the first couple of weeks after my children were born when my breasts were very heavy and full of milk. Some women can get away with wearing no bra at any time, including when they are breastfeeding, while others prefer to wear one even at night, as well as during the day, to prevent stretch marks and drooping boobs. Just do whatever makes you feel most comfortable. If you do choose to wear a bra, buy one with wide shoulder straps. If you plan to breastfeed, choose a bra that opens at the front. You will probably need to buy several, in gradually increasing sizes. Most large chemist's shops stock special maternity bras which are fairly well upholstered without being too unsightly or bulky, and which have a flap over the front for breastfeeding.

Shoes are another important item of clothing. Because your posture and sense of balance change during pregnancy, as the bump on your front enlarges, it is important to wear the right kind of shoes. Basically, this just means wearing shoes with a low, flat heel, so that you are not put off balance when you walk, or made to tilt your pelvis forward by the height of a heel. You shouldn't have any trouble finding low-heeled shoes in the shops; there are plenty of very fashionable ones around, as well as low-heeled boots and sandals. Low court shoes and espadrilles are particularly comfortable, practical and attractive. Avoid sling-backs or shoes with ankle straps which could affect the circulation, since your ankles can swell during pregnancy. Look out for flat pumps, slip-ons and flattie sandals. Flat laced shoes and bar shoes are also good. There are many different styles and colours to choose from, so you shouldn't have any difficulty finding something you like.

Skin

The quality of your skin is an indication of the health of your body. Its colour and texture are clues to your well-being. During pregnancy you want to look your best, and your skin is one of the first things to consider. Your skin is the foundation for good looks – if your complexion is healthy and silky-looking it sets your whole face aglow and is the basis upon which you can build your cosmetic beauty – so it is important to take care of your skin, in order to make the best of it. Luckily for many women, pregnancy brings with it a 'blooming' effect which makes the skin look radiant, glowing and healthy. This is the time to make the most of what you've got, and to pamper yourself and your skin. Skin is a living organ, just like any other organ of the body, and it needs the correct nourishment and feeding in order to function properly. Skin reacts to changes and extremes of temperature such as central heating, sun or cold winds, so it needs to be protected from these with moisturizers and sun lotions, especially during pregnancy when the skin may be extra sensitive. Skin needs to be cleansed and washed to remove the leftover make-up, dirt or chemicals from the atmosphere that build up on it during the day.

It is helpful to know how the skin is built and how it works so that you can take appropriate action to keep it in good condition. In fact the skin is a very complicated organ. It is made up of many different layers, and contains many other structures, such as sweat glands and hair follicles. The layers are grouped together to form the two major parts of the skin, the *epidermis* and the *dermis*.

The epidermis is the top, superficial part of the skin. It can be fairly thin and delicate in certain parts of the body, such as the face and neck, or it can become hardened and thickened in other areas, such as the palms of the hands and the soles of the feet. The surface layer of the epidermis is made up from dead cells, which form a tough, outer coat. As time goes by these dead cells are replaced by other dying cells, and the top layer gradually sloughs off and flakes away. It is this action which we try to regulate, by using creams and moisturizers so that our surface skin stays smooth and supple.

The dermis is much thicker than the epidermis, and is the part of the skin which holds most of the other structures, such as the hair follicles. There is very little you can do from the outside to affect the dermis, but if you want to take skin care to its logical conclusion you can make sure you eat a varied and balanced diet of fresh foods, because the dermis is 'fed' with the nutrients it needs by tiny blood vessels called capillaries, and the quality of the blood in your veins depends greatly on the food you eat. If you follow a varied, natural diet, as described in Chapter 4, you will be helping your skin to be healthy as well as the rest of your body. Various different structures are distributed throughout the dermis, including many very fine blood vessels which form a capillary network supplying blood to the roots of the hair, the sebaceous glands and the sweat glands. There is also a fine network of lymphatic capillaries which supply nutrients to the upper layers of the skin. Many touch-sensitive organs are also found in the dermis – these give us our sense of touch and are sensitive to changes in temperature, pressure and stimulation. Sweat glands are found in the dermis, and these are part of the mechanism by which the body loses excess water, helping to maintain the correct body temperature. Hair follicles are found in the dermis all over the body, except in the soles of the feet, the palms of the hands and the mouth. A sebaceous gland is found in each hair follicle shaft; these produce sebum, which lubricates the hair and keeps the outer layer of skin supple. By each hair shaft there is also a special muscle called the *arrector pili*, which comes into action when the skin becomes cold, raising the hair and causing goose pimples.

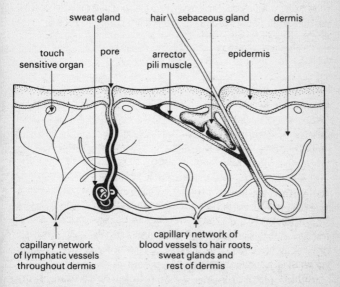

Fig. 11. The components of the skin.

How your skin changes during pregnancy

During pregnancy the skin undergoes changes, and may feel and look different. This does not happen in one predictable way for all women, however – it depends on the individual. Generally speaking, though, dry skin tends to become drier and flakier, while oily skin becomes more oily. The majority of women certainly find that their skin sweats more when they are pregnant, not only in the usual places but also on the face, the palms of the hands, the feet and the legs. In fact, during pregnancy the production of sweat seems noticeably to increase over the whole area of skin on the body. This does not really matter, but it does necessitate extra baths or showers and more frequent washing. For most mothers-to-be this should not pose much of a problem, except where washing facilities are limited. If you are in the habit of wearing a lot of make-up, you may have to wash it off and re-apply it during the day if too much sweat disturbs it. Try to keep as cool as possible by wearing cool, absorbent, cotton clothes that allow your skin to breathe. Wash frequently, and don't over-exert yourself.

Facial skin

Follow a regular skin care routine for your face and neck, twice a day if you can manage it. Start by using a good cleansing cream to remove make-up, surface grime and any oiliness, then remove the cleanser with warm water and dry your skin. Splash ice-cold water on to your face to close the pores and tone the skin – this will give just as good a result as an expensive toning liquid, although you can use the latter if you prefer. Dry your skin and then apply a moisturizer. Use a light moisturizer if your skin tends to be oily, a richer one if your skin is dry and flaky. If you follow this skin care routine once or twice a day, it will prevent your pores getting clogged up with extra sweat.

Some women find that their skin becomes much more sensitive during pregnancy. If any itching or irritation occurs, ask your doctor's advice. If you find wearing your normal make-up uncomfortable because of extra sensitivity, try using one of the non-allergic ranges, or use eye make-up specially made for contact lens wearers, available from most opticians. These mascaras and powder eyeshadows are smudge-proof and non-flaky, and are less likely to irritate the skin and the eyes. Face packs are also a good idea during pregnancy, since they draw out and soak up perspiration and impurities from the skin, leaving it smooth, supple and tightened. When the face pack is removed a layer of dead cells is removed with it, leaving the skin silky-soft and glowing. Try to use a face pack at least once a week during pregnancy, to stop the build-up of grime – it will be cooling and refreshing too. Leave the face pack on for 10–20 minutes or until it begins to dry around the edges. Wash it off with warm water, dry the skin, then moisturize.

During the later stages of pregnancy, a few women notice an increase in pigmentation of the skin, particularly on the face, although it can also affect the breasts and tummy. This extra pigmentation is actually quite unusual. On the face it consists of a slight darkening of the skin covering the nose and cheeks. It looks a bit like a rash, but does not itch. There is nothing that can be done about it except to wait until the baby is born, when it will probably disappear of its own accord fairly quickly. Sometimes freckles and moles on the skin also darken, and it is not unusual for the colour of the nipples to darken too, and for the area of nipple to increase. All these changes in pigment seem to be more noticeable in brunettes and those who have darker complexions to begin with – redheads and blondes seem to suffer less from this particular side effect.

Stretchmarks

The skin on the rest of the body also needs special attention during pregnancy. Many pregnant women complain of stretchmarks on their enlarging stomachs, hips, breasts and thighs. These are red or pink streaks in the skin, and are caused when the skin is stretched beyond its normal elasticity. After the baby is born the stretchmarks gradually fade to a silvery-grey colour, but they never disappear altogether. If you want to try to avoid stretchmarks while your baby is growing and your figure is expanding, the best preventive measure of all is to try to limit your weight gain to a reasonable level (i.e. not more than 2 stone over the whole pregnancy) so that the skin does not have to stretch more than is necessary. Increased hormone levels are also thought to be partially responsible for stretchmarks in some cases, and while there are a number of expensive creams and oils made specially for mothers-to-be, there is little evidence that these have any real effect. It is unlikely that oiling the top layer of your skin will prevent it from succumbing to stretchmarks, which are, after all, due to excess stretching of the underlying tissues and not of the upper layer of skin itself, although it will help to keep your skin supple and stop it from drying out. By all means use oil and creams on your tummy to keep your skin well moisturized and smooth, but don't expect any miracles. You don't need to buy costly maternity creams – any type of cream will do. If you are prone to stretchmarks there is not much you can do to avoid them except to limit your weight gain. If you are lucky, and also manage to keep your weight at a reasonable level, you may find that they never appear.

Breasts are a slightly different matter. Stretchmarks on the breasts can be made worse if a woman has very large, heavy or sagging breasts. If your breasts increase dramatically in size when you first become pregnant, you will benefit from wearing a well-fitting, supportive bra. This will help to prevent your breasts sagging and stretching too much, thereby avoiding stretchmarks. If you don't notice much change in the size of your breasts, you will probably be all right without a bra at all. Just do whatever makes you feel most comfortable.

Sunbathing

The action of sunlight on the skin causes Vitamin D to be formed for use in the body. For this reason a little sunbathing during pregnancy is a good idea. However, care should be taken not to over-expose the body to very hot, bright sunlight when you are pregnant, because you may find that your skin is more sensitive at this time and cannot tolerate the same level of sun-tanning as was previously possible. Take care to use plenty of sun lotion if you do sunbathe, since you may find you are much more susceptible to burning.

Hair

Some women find that their hair looks its best during pregnancy, becoming glossy, lustrous, thick and healthy-looking. Others find that it becomes inexplicably dry, breaking and splitting much too easily. Whatever the state of your hair during pregnancy, the best beauty treatment you can give it is to use a very mild, gentle shampoo and follow a good diet. The visible hair on your head is quite dead, but the root of each hair is alive and is nourished and grows by using the nutrients from the food you eat. The base of the hair follicle where the hair root nestles is fed with nutrients by a capillary network of tiny blood vessels.

Teeth

It is extremely important to take good care of your teeth during pregnancy, because at this time your gums are more susceptible to bleeding and infection, making it more likely that your teeth will decay too. Right at the beginning of pregnancy your gums soften and are more prone to inflammation. As a result your gums can be more easily damaged by hard pieces of food, and, once damaged, infection can quickly set in. While you are pregnant this can happen most easily where the gum meets a tooth – a damaged gum quickly leads to a damaged and decaying tooth, so careful brushing and mouth hygiene are essential. If your gums start to bleed, consult your dentist as soon as possible. Dentists repair damaged teeth, but it is far better to prevent the damage occurring in the first place by careful diet and adequate maintenance of teeth.

Teeth and gums are attacked by plaque, which is a layer of bacteria that grows on both the teeth and the gums. If you eat a lot of sugary foods you will increase the amount of plaque growing on your teeth, since the bacteria in plaque feed on sugar. If you eat less sugar the bacteria won't get such a good opportunity to grow and multiply. If plaque is left to grow indefinitely and the teeth are not brushed regularly, the plaque will start to eat into the enamel surface of the tooth. If this is allowed to continue, the tooth will keep on decaying until it affects the nerve inside, causing toothache. Brushing your teeth once or twice a day is normally enough to keep plaque at bay, but when you are pregnant it is a good idea to brush your teeth after every meal, to make sure the plaque does not have a chance to get a hold on your teeth while they are in a more delicate condition. Do make sure you use a *soft* brush for your teeth while you are pregnant. Too hard a bristle will damage your gums instead of stimulating and cleaning them. A brush with a small head is best, so that you can reach all the awkward corners and surfaces of the teeth. Renew your toothbrush when the bristles start to look droopy, or flat, or begin to splay out. Use a fluoride toothpaste for extra protection. If you are not sure whether you are succeeding in brushing away all the plaque, try using some disclosing tablets or liquid, which dye the plaque red or pink. When all the colour has been brushed away, you will be sure that all the plaque has gone. It is especially important during pregnancy to remove any tiny pieces of food that get stuck between your teeth, as they will irritate the gums – use dental floss or dental sticks for this.

Visit your dentist as soon as you know you are pregnant. Tell him of your pregnancy, and continue to visit him regularly during the nine months. Take additional care of your teeth by eating fewer sugary items in your diet. Don't forget that teeth were designed with chewing in mind, so don't eat only soft, mushy foods but include raw vegetables and crunchy fruit in your daily diet to get your teeth working properly. Wholewheat products are more chewy than their processed, white alternatives. A stick of raw carrot or celery or a crunchy apple is better than a sweet snack and will use your teeth for the purpose for which they were designed – chewing, biting, crunching and grinding.

Calcium tablets are sometimes prescribed during pregnancy, and some people think that this is to protect the mother's teeth. However, this is not so. Extra calcium is given to protect the mother's bones only, not the teeth, from loss of calcium. If there is not enough calcium in the mother's diet to form the baby's bones and teeth in the uterus it will 'steal' some from its mother's bones, making them brittle, but this does not happen in the same way with the mother's teeth, and the teeth themselves are unlikely to soften, only the gums. Rather than taking tablets, the best way to ensure an adequate calcium intake is to drink a pint of milk each day. There is an old wives' tale which says that for every baby you carry you will lose a tooth, but this need not be so if you take adequate care and brush your teeth properly. Remember that your gums are more sensitive and prone to decay during pregnancy, so give them the attention they deserve and you need not suffer any adverse effects.

Nails

Your fingernails and toenails are made from skin which has been modified and hardened to form a protective covering for the sensitive ends of the fingers and toes. The root of the nail is embedded in a fold of the skin and is covered by the cuticle. Many women find that when they are pregnant their nails become more brittle and flaky, splitting or breaking more easily, so you may need extra protection during this time. Try rubbing oil or moisturizing cream frequently into the base of the nails, to keep the cuticle soft and to give the nails a natural shine. Massage it in every day for the best results. Wear protective gloves for gardening, and use rubber gloves for messy jobs and for those that involve the use of strong soaps, detergents or bleach, as these will dry the nails out even further. If your nails become very weak you can buy some nail hardener, which is painted on and dries into a protective coat on top of the existing nail. Keep brittle nails short, so that they have less opportunity to snap or break.

Posture

Good posture is essential in pregnancy because as the baby grows your pelvis tends to tilt forward, making your lower back more arched and causing you to stick your bottom out. If you lack good posture before you become pregnant you may find that these postural effects of pregnancy make you very uncomfortable, giving you backache and overstretching the muscles of your abdomen. By the end of your pregnancy you will have altered your normal walk to help compensate for the effects of your different posture, giving you the characteristic waddle of the heavily pregnant lady. If you can learn to stand straighter, keep your bottom tucked in, and use your abdominal muscles instead of just letting them go, you will benefit by feeling better, looking better, and suffering less from backache and tiredness. There is a lot to be said for reviewing your posture long before you even conceive your baby, correcting it if necessary so that you will be on the right track from the very start. Then when you do become pregnant and the bump on your front starts to enlarge enough to put you slightly off your balance, you will be aware of any postural changes and will know how to compensate for them. The muscles you will need to counteract the effects of the pregnant posture will already be toned up and strong enough to reduce the likelihood of severe backache and diminish the possibility of you losing your sense of balance too drastically.

Good posture is simply a matter of balance of the different parts of the body – the weight should be evenly distributed down your spine to your hips, knees and feet. Gravity has a constant effect on the body, pulling you down to the ground, and you resist the force of gravity by using your muscles to hold yourself erect. If you allow some of these muscles to slacken, other muscles will tighten to compensate and the alignment of your body will change, resulting in bad posture and putting strain on your back and other parts of your body. In the extreme, bad posture can mean that your internal organs are squashed unnaturally downwards or sideways and therefore may not work efficiently. Bad posture is almost certain to give you backache, disturb your coordination, affect the flexibility of your body and make you lose your balance. So it is obviously important to try to correct a sagging posture and any figure faults when you are pregnant (or beforehand if possible), so that you are spared any further stress and strain on your body due to the uneven distribution of weight that pregnancy inevitably brings.

A good posture for standing

To visualize what a good standing posture should be, try to imagine a straight, vertical line running through your body at 90 degrees to the ground you are standing on. The line should start just behind your ear, then go down through the shoulder joint, just behind the hip joint, just in front of the knee joint, and finish between the heel and the ball of the foot. To add to the efficiency of this stance, think about your muscles too. Pull your tummy muscles in, tuck your bottom in (don't stick it out, it's most unattractive), and try to keep your back fairly straight (no gaping hollows, please). It is obviously difficult to see a side view of yourself, so ask someone to help you sort out your posture faults (most of us have some), using the illustration and comments here. If you get your posture correct before conceiving, you probably won't suffer too much when your lump starts to grow larger and threatens to alter your sense of balance. Keep practising good posture whenever you find yourself standing around – in a bus queue, at the kitchen sink, at the supermarket checkout, peeling the vegetables, etc. – and you will soon get to the stage where it becomes automatic. Good posture

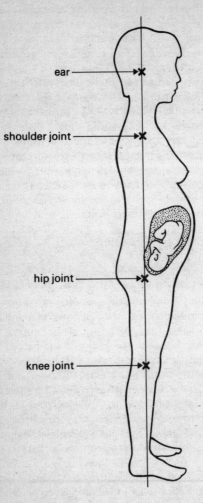

Fig. 12. Good posture.

makes you look more attractive too, and helps to keep your pregnancy invisible for longer.

Walking

Your normal centre of gravity should be somewhere around your sacral vertebrae (the bones at the base of your spine), which are fused together and collectively called the sacrum. When you move forward to walk, the movement should start from this centre of gravity. Try to keep your feet parallel and to swing your legs from the hip. At the same time, remember to keep your tummy pulled in and your bottom tucked under, keeping your back fairly flat, as before.

Sitting

When you sit in a chair, try not to let your back slouch into a rounded shape or let your shoulders droop forward. Your lower back area should have good support, and should be neither too rounded (convex) nor too hollowed (concave). If you don't seem to fit properly into your chairs at home, place a cushion behind your lower back for extra support.

Your shoes are important too

The sort of shoes you wear can make a difference to your overall posture. If you wear high heels during pregnancy this will accentuate the forward tilting of the pelvis, which is undesirable. So make low heels and flat shoes the rule. Your feet are very important during pregnancy because they have to take the strain and carry all the extra weight you acquire. This puts an increased strain on the arches of the feet, so you should wear well-fitting, comfortable shoes with plenty of room all round your toes. Your feet may spread while you are pregnant, because of the extra weight, and you may even need to buy shoes half a size larger than your normal size.

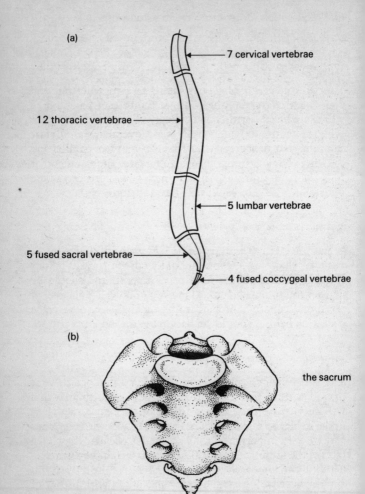

(a)

7 cervical vertebrae

12 thoracic vertebrae

5 lumbar vertebrae

5 fused sacral vertebrae

4 fused coccygeal vertebrae

(b)

the sacrum

Fig. 13. (a) The curves and vertebrae of the spine. (b) The sacrum.

Bending down, picking up, reaching up and carrying

Bending down: During pregnancy, and indeed at any other time, the accent is on bending *down* and not bending over. To bend down to the floor, put one foot forward ahead of the other and bend your knees so that your body is lowered smoothly and steadily, keeping your spine erect. As your body is lowered down, lift the heel of the foot that is at the back so that your leg is resting on the ball of your foot and your toes.

Picking up: Use the bending position, above, for picking objects up, and keep your spine erect as you stand up.

Reaching up: Keep your feet apart to help you keep your balance properly. If you want to reach a very high shelf above your head, it's best to use some steps or a stool. Avoid standing on tiptoe to reach high objects, as you could lose your balance and topple over.

Carrying: It is said that the best place to carry a load is on top of your head. Naturally you cannot visualize yourself walking down the high street in all your pregnant glory with a bundle of shopping balanced on top of your head, so compromise by making sure you always carry it in two evenly weighted bags, one in each hand. This way all the weight will not be uncomfortably on one side, making you walk in a lopsided manner. Alternatively, carry the load in front of you in your outstretched arms, keeping the load in the middle, not resting on one side or the other.

The psychological changes

During pregnancy your body is obviously changing, growing and maturing, but what about your state of mind and your mental attitudes and thought processes? Although many mothers-to-be don't realize it, they undergo great psychological changes and growth during pregnancy. These changes are not so apparent as the bump on your front, but nevertheless they are very important, and if a woman is aware of them she will be better able to cope with what might otherwise be interpreted as odd, unreasonable changes in her character and moods.

While you are pregnant the spotlight falls on you – you are in the limelight, you are the important figure whom friends and neighbours ask after. After your baby is born you won't have much time to think about yourself, at least in the short term, and the baby will be the centre of everyone's attention and admiration. You will be left rather in the background. This is something many mothers do not anticipate, but it is vitally important to accept the fact that you will soon have to adjust your role from 'pregnant wife' to 'mother', and also to understand just what this entails in terms of your time and energy. Motherhood is no easy option, it takes dedication and self-sacrifice to do the job well. You are bound to experience problems and troubles (although they won't last for ever) as well as joys. Preparing for this in advance will alleviate the symptoms and help you to adjust more easily, so use your nine months of pregnancy to plan ahead and think about the likely stresses and problems of motherhood. Every woman reacts to the experience of birth with different emotions and feelings. Apart from feelings of elation and fulfilment, you may also suffer from extreme tiredness, lassitude, fits of crying, and sometimes a sense of utter helplessness and inability to cope. If you are prepared for this you won't be in such a state of shock when it happens. You will know that it is to be expected and that it will eventually pass, you will know that it is possible to get through this period and be able to cope. Use your pregnancy as a time to acknowledge the difficulties to come and face them with a positive mind.

Right from the start of your pregnancy you will sometimes feel your moods and emotions swing from one extreme to the other as your hormones play havoc with your sense of emotional stability. You may find you sometimes become unavoidably dozy and vague or forgetful, while at other times you are bad-tempered or hot-headed. There may be days when you just can't seem to stop crying, or there may be times when you just want to sleep for hours and hours. Of course you may not suffer from any of these symptoms, or they may be so slight that you are not even aware of them, but for most of us they are common occurrences in pregnancy and after the birth. If you encounter these swings of mood and emotion and don't understand why they happen, it can make you feel even worse. For instance, if you feel depressed and weepy one morning and don't know why, you may find that the feeling becomes a desperately unhappy, painful self-criticism, and perhaps suspect yourself of cracking up. Remember that these moods are normal – they happen to most, if not all, pregnant women to some degree.

Nobody really knows what causes this reaction in pregnancy. It almost certainly has something to do with hormone levels, but I believe it also relates strongly to the new mother-role a woman faces. She has to continue coming to terms with her new role after the baby is born, and something like ten out of every twelve women experience the 'baby blues', or a time of unexplained moodiness and emotional distress a few days after giving birth. Most women come to terms with their new role fairly quickly. It is probably best to give in to the weepy, helpless feelings, knowing that they are only transitory, and then get on with living the rest of your life. Life is rarely completely easy; things don't just fall into place and go as smoothly as you might suppose from watching films or reading magazines, but knowing that your feelings are normal and understandable, and that you are not a freak or a failure for letting go, makes it all bearable. Women expect to *look* different physically during pregnancy, they know that their shape, weight and size will change dramatically, and because the body cannot be separated from the mind they should be prepared to *feel* different mentally as well.

6

Minor Ailments and How to Cope with Them

During pregnancy many physical changes occur, and also a lot of minor discomforts, such as morning sickness and heartburn. While most of these are not actually dangerous, and do not put either the mother or the baby in jeopardy, they can still be very uncomfortable and tedious. It is quite likely that you will meet one or two of these minor ailments as your pregnancy progresses, although some lucky women never encounter any at all. Many of these minor symptoms of pregnancy can be avoided, or at least made less severe, by simple means such as a modified diet, and need no treatment from your doctor. Other more serious problems, such as oedema or high blood pressure, will always need expert attention. The following pages describe the ailments you may expect to come across during your pregnancy, and give advice on how to deal with them. If, however, you are in any doubt about your symptoms, or are worried that your pregnancy is not progressing normally, you should consult your doctor.

Anaemia

When you first visit your antenatal clinic you will be asked to give a small sample of blood so that certain tests can be carried out. These tests include identifying your blood group and rhesus factor, and making a haemoglobin count. The test for haemoglobin is concerned with measuring the level of iron in your blood, to see if you are, or are likely to become, anaemic while you are pregnant. Haemoglobin is the protein in the red blood cells, and is the means by which oxygen is conveyed from the lungs to the rest of the cells in the body, including the baby in the womb. If there is not enough haemoglobin in the mother's blood, there may not be enough oxygen reaching the baby for optimum growth and development. As the baby needs more and more oxygen and nutrients from its mother's blood as it grows larger and more mature, the haemoglobin count in the mother's blood can fall to an anaemic level at any time during her pregnancy, which is why blood tests are carried out periodically, throughout the nine months. The tell-tale signs of anaemia in the mother include a general lethargy and lack of energy. She may constantly feel tired out and exhausted, irritable, bad-tempered and depressed, generally weak and overworked, although physically she may be doing very little. It is necessary to use a blood test to confirm a diagnosis of anaemia, because for some women these symptoms can also be due to the start of pregnancy itself, and the two causes of similar symptoms should not be confused. Anaemic women often look very pale and drawn too, with a greyish, whitish look to the skin.

The treatment of anaemia is quite simple, and just involves the mother increasing her daily intake of iron until the required level of haemoglobin in the blood is reached. This can be accomplished either by a change of diet, or by taking iron tablets, or both. If you are planning to conceive in the near future, you can prepare yourself by taking a course of iron tablets, available from a chemist. You can also watch your diet, making sure you eat plenty of iron-rich foods – liver and other offal, red meat, wholewheat bread and flour, and green vegetables, for example dark green cabbage, spring greens, curly kale, broccoli, mustard and cress, parsley and watercress. Spinach has a high iron content too, but unfortunately most of it cannot be used by the body because other substances in the spinach block the absorption of iron into the blood. Not all the iron eaten in any food can be fully absorbed into the blood, so the recommended intake of iron for a pregnant woman (15 mg per day) is more than the actual minimum requirements to allow for some wastage.

It must also be said that if you avoid putting on too much

weight during your pregnancy, the less blood and therefore the less haemoglobin you will need to sustain your body. Extra unnecessary weight needs extra blood to supply it with oxygen and other nutrients, overworking all the mechanisms of the body, which is yet another good reason and incentive to keep your weight gain at or below 2 stone during your pregnancy.

Appetite control

Two extremes of this problem can arise during pregnancy. The first usually occurs in the earlier weeks of pregnancy, when you may be suffering from morning sickness and general tiredness which can result in poor eating habits and an unbalanced diet. The second is concerned with eating too much, owing to an enormous increase in appetite and hunger. This is probably partly a result of increased levels of hormones in pregnancy, but is also exaggerated by boredom and inactive monotony.

Counteracting a poor appetite: Special care needs to be taken during the first twelve weeks of pregnancy to ensure that you have a balanced, healthy diet. Remember that for the foetus this is the most crucial, vital time, when all the important parts of its body are growing and developing and it needs plenty of nutrients to prosper. If you suffer from loss of appetite at this time, just try to make sure that what little you do eat is the right sort of 'building' material for the baby. Concentrate on eating food rich in protein, vitamins and minerals and try to avoid sugary, sweet things. If you can't face cooking anything because of nausea, try eating uncooked foods such as salads, pick and choose from a selection of different cheeses with biscuits, or try sandwiches or a bowl of muesli. Don't worry about conventional mealtimes when you are feeling like this – if you fancy a bowl of muesli for your evening meal that's excellent. The time when you eat your meals is less important than what goes into them. If you can't eat anything solid at all, try pepping up your drinks with some added goodness. Try whisking up nutritious milk shakes in a liquidizer, adding an egg, a banana and some honey or malt extract. You could use yogurt for the base instead of milk. If you really can't face eating anything at all, and if a total lack of appetite continues for more than a couple of days, consult your doctor.

Counteracting an over-zealous appetite: This is a bit more difficult to curb, since the remedy lies in strong will and perseverance and during pregnancy for various reasons these may be elusive qualities where food is concerned. Whatever the cause, many women certainly find that while they are pregnant they are continually hungry and cannot easily satiate their ravenous appetites. The old saying about 'eating for two' may stem from this excessive hunger in pregnancy, but desire should not be confused with necessity. You do not *need* to eat that much, and it is a matter of balancing your intake of food against your calorific requirements if you are to avoid excess weight. An expectant mother who constantly over-eats risks putting on far too much weight, and this increases the likelihood of oedema, high blood pressure, or a variety of other problems connected with overweight. It also looks most unattractive, and feels unpleasant. If you find that your appetite increases abnormally, do your very best to control it. Try to eat more fresh fruit and vegetables and fewer sugary items. Try to cultivate your taste to prefer the less calorific foods. Go for fibre-rich foods which will help to fill you up and keep you satisfied until the next meal. Be strict about mealtimes, and don't nibble in between. Try to chew your food more slowly, and avoid binges. You may have a hard battle to stay on the right side of the dreaded daily calorie total, but do persevere, please, it's worth the effort to stay slim. I know from experience just how difficult it can be, but I can also assure you that the results are well worth the extra effort. If you are not sure what your daily calorie intake adds up to, make a list of everything you eat (weighing each portion of food) and at the end of the day add up the total, using the calorie guide at the end of this book. You may have a nasty shock, as you could be overdoing it without realizing it. While you are pregnant you should not eat more than

2,400 calories per day *at the very most*, and I think this is actually rather generous – for most of us 2,000 calories is plenty even during pregnancy. If you find it difficult to restrict your calories to around 2,000 per day while you are pregnant, try to take your mind off food by getting involved in something else between meals. Get out and about, do some gentle gardening, take a walk, read a good book (or better still, write one). Make yourself a new dress or knit a jumper. Keep busy, do whatever you enjoy, get moving, however gently, and keep both your body and your mind active. Don't sit around the house all day doing nothing but eating. Food should not be a compensation for loneliness or boredom. Make contact with some other expectant mothers at your local antenatal clinic – you will find you are not the only one with an adventurous appetite. Ask one or two others home to discuss ways of coping with it over a cup of tea (but not over a packet of biscuits).

Backache

The weight gained during pregnancy causes extra strain on the joints and on the parts of the body that support your body weight. This in turn alters your posture, causing even more strain on your back and supportive muscles. The best treatment for backache in pregnancy is to concentrate on realigning your body by standing and sitting correctly. Avoid slouching in chairs or standing lopsidedly or awkwardly while you are pregnant (see 'Posture', pp. 116–21). It is worth practising a good posture, and trying to hold your tummy in and keep your bottom tucked under, because it will make such a difference to your visual appearance as well as helping to relieve your backache. It may not be easy if you have been used to slouching about for years, but once you have learned the technique of standing up straight again and keeping a good posture, you will soon find that it becomes second nature to you and you will no longer need to think consciously about holding yourself erect. Backache can also be relieved by getting plenty of rest when you need it. Try not to stand for long periods of time; for example, sit on a kitchen stool while preparing vegetables. Try to arrange your timetable so that you can sit and rest in a comfortable chair for half an hour, mid morning and mid afternoon. When you sit down in an armchair, support your lower back with a cushion to keep the natural curve of the spine and eliminate a rounded back. Massage may also help to relieve an aching back (husbands can help here), as will a hot water bottle. Excess weight will increase back strain, so try to keep your weight gain at a reasonable level.

Breathlessness

Breathlessness in pregnancy is caused when the growing womb pushes the abdomen upwards, forcing the lungs into a squashed shape which cannot completely fill with air as easily as usual. This symptom usually becomes more pronounced later on in pregnancy, when the womb is at its largest. You may find yourself gasping for air, sighing deeply, or panting and out of breath after climbing a flight of stairs. The symptoms often become worse when you lie down, as the baby in your womb then falls back on to your abdominal organs more acutely, leaving even less space for your lungs. Make sure you don't overwork yourself if you find that you are easily becoming breathless while you are pregnant. It is important that you take things easy and do not attempt to do anything you know to be impossible in your present state. Know your physical limits and don't overstep them. Try to keep a good posture, stand up straight, and sit upright so that your lungs have as much space as you can give them, despite the lump. If you find that the breathlessness becomes worse at night, prop yourself up in bed with some extra pillows or cushions and sleep in a sitting position rather than lying down. (This will also help to counteract heartburn.)

Coughs and colds

Most people will catch at least one cold during the course of nine months, especially if there are other children in the family who are at school, where they are likely to catch the occasional infection and bring it home. The symptoms of a cold, coupled with morning sickness and/or other symptoms of pregnancy, will probably make you feel particularly miserable. Although a cold during pregnancy will not affect your baby in any way, it will make you feel absolutely ghastly and may hit you harder than a cold normally would. If possible, retreat to bed with a hot water bottle until you are over the worst. Try to stay out of contact with other expectant mothers while you are still infectious. If you suffer repeatedly from diarrhoea or sickness with a cold for more than a day or two, you should consult your doctor. If you develop a very bad cough, consult your doctor before taking any cough medicine. Try to avoid contact with anyone who is suffering from a cold during the weeks leading up to your expected confinement. You should try to avoid having a cold while you are in labour.

Constipation

Because of extra progesterone in the blood during pregnancy the muscle tone of the lower digestive organs is lowered, and this very often results in constipation. This can happen right at the beginning of pregnancy and can carry on throughout the whole nine months. If you want to help yourself there is no need to use laxatives – there is a much gentler and more effective dietary way of dealing with constipation. First you can increase the amount of water you consume each day, as more liquid makes the stools softer and therefore helps eliminate the problem. Try to drink about four pints of liquid each day. Avoid fizzy, sweetened drinks, and use fresh fruit juices, tea, herb teas or just plain water instead. Herb teas are especially good – they taste lovely and leave your mouth tasting sweet and fresh, unlike conventional tea and coffee. As an added bonus they contain no calories whatsoever –

perfect! The second dietary step you can take is to make sure that you eat plenty of fibre in your diet. Use wholewheat products whenever you can – wholewheat bread, wholewheat pasta, etc. Leave the skins on your potatoes and other cooked vegetables. Eat wholegrain muesli for breakfast. If the problem still persists, try sprinkling a tablespoonful of bran on your breakfast cereal each day. This extra fibre is not digested like other food but passes straight through you. By the time it has reached your gut it will have absorbed lots of extra water, thus providing more bulk in the stools and making them softer and easier to get rid of. If you don't fancy bran with your breakfast, add it to soups, gravies, meat loaves or pies instead. Never take laxatives in pregnancy unless your doctor prescribes them.

Cramp

Cramp in the lower legs often occurs during the night, and it can be sufficiently painful to wake you from a deep sleep. It can happen during the day too. The calf muscles contract into a lumpy knot, and the muscle has to be smoothed out again to relieve the pain. The best method of dealing with cramp is forcibly to extend the muscle back again by pulling your foot upwards. Push your ankle joint upwards and bend your toes up so that the muscle straightens out again. Massaging the muscle at the same time also helps; stroke it firmly or knead it with the palm of your hand or your knuckles. In the past it was mistakenly thought that all cramp is caused by a lack of salt in the diet. It is now known that this is in fact quite rare, and that cramp is more likely to be caused by lack of calcium. Pregnant women should try to avoid taking too much extra salt because it can encourage the retention of water in the body, something to avoid during pregnancy. Instead take calcium tablets or eat plenty of calcium-rich foods to help prevent it happening again. Cramp in the lower legs can also be caused by varicose veins. If you continue to suffer from severe cramp, consult your doctor.

Cystitis

This is a very common complaint, and some women seem to be more prone to it during pregnancy. Cystitis is an infection of the urinary tract which causes inflammation of the bladder and of the urethra, the pipe through which the urine is passed to the outside. The first symptom is usually a desire to pass water much more frequently than normal, sometimes only minutes after having already done so. Most of the time, although you may feel absolutely desperate to reach the lavatory, you won't be able to pass much urine at all once you get there, maybe only a little trickle, or none at all. This is coupled with an acute sensation of burning or stinging when you do manage to pass some urine, however little, and the urine itself may look a very dark yellow colour, much darker than normal, and in extreme cases may have streaks of blood in it. This kind of infection is very easily caused in women because of the female anatomy: because the openings to the vagina, urethra and anus are all very close together, germs which may be harmless in the bowel can very easily get transmitted to the urethra and vagina. It is important to consult your doctor as soon as possible if you have an attack of cystitis, because if it is left untreated the infection can travel up to the kidneys and this is much more painful and more dangerous. Cystitis is very easily treated, once diagnosed, and a course of antibiotics will soon get rid of the infection. To relieve the symptoms of cystitis immediately (if it hits you in the middle of the night), drink half a pint of water every half an hour to dilute the strength of the urine and to help flush the infection through before it has a chance to become established and really take a hold. Any watery liquid will do, for example weak tea or herb tea, but avoid strong tea or coffee. Plain water is best, if you can drink large quantities of it without getting bored with the taste. Some people find it helpful to take a teaspoonful of bicarbonate of soda dissolved in water, repeated at hourly intervals, as this helps to make the urine less acidic and therefore less painful when excreted.

If you have suffered from cystitis several times before, and think you may be prone to developing the infection again, there are two things you can do to lessen the likelihood of an attack. First, make sure you drink plenty of watery liquids every day (up to four pints if you can manage it); this will help to flush urine through your system more quickly, taking with it any lingering germs before they get a chance to multiply. Second, make an effort to be extra hygienic and wash your genitals once or twice a day. Use a mild soap or just plain water. Don't use any strong soap solutions or anything with harsh chemicals. Start at the front and work backwards, to prevent any germs from the anus getting near the urethral opening.

Diarrhoea

Diarrhoea sometimes occurs in early pregnancy, and should be reported to your doctor if it persists for more than a day or two. Iron tablets can cause diarrhoea in some women, and in this case the problem can usually be remedied simply by changing to another brand of iron pill. During the remainder of pregnancy the problem is more likely to be constipation, although some women do report having diarrhoea during the early stages of labour, probably due to the hormones which cause labour to start.

Fainting and dizziness

Many women complain of dizziness and a feeling of faintness when they first become pregnant, and this sometimes continues through the first twelve weeks of pregnancy. For some women the symptoms are severe enough for them actually to lose consciousness for a moment or two. This is not harmful to the growing baby or to the mother, except that the mother may injure herself if she falls to the ground in a faint. Fainting and dizziness are caused by a lowering of the blood pressure, so that not enough blood and oxygen reach the brain. Once fainting has occurred and you have fallen to the ground, the blood is able to reach your brain more easily again, because your heart no longer needs to pump blood upwards to your head, and the dizziness leaves you. The only preventive measure you can take is to make sure you don't stand still for long periods of time but keep on the move, so that your blood is encouraged to keep pumping around at an adequate pace. Keep out of situations you find claustrophobic, such as stuffy cinemas and hot, crowded shops, and wear loose, cool clothes. If you feel faint at any time, head for the nearest chair or flat surface and sit or lie down. Try to get out into the fresh air and breathe deeply. If necessary, put your head down between your knees until you recover. Some situations, such as standing up when getting out of a very hot bath, can also make you feel lightheaded, and the same effect can happen even if you just stand up too quickly after sitting still for a while. If you drive, take extra care if you find you suffer from dizziness. If you feel at all faint or giddy while driving, pull over and stop until the symptoms recede.

Flatulence

Flatulence, which is often euphemistically called 'wind', is a problem that few people like to admit to. However, it is a fact that in early pregnancy it can be a nuisance. Although it is not harmful, it can be extremely embarrassing. If you are a sufferer, don't eat gaseous foods or drink fizzy drinks, and don't eat any beans, peas or over-rich foods. If the problem still persists you could try to cultivate the art of burping, in an effort to remove any excess air from the stomach before it has a chance to enter the gut.

Food cravings

Serious, uncontrollable cravings to eat certain foods or even coal or soil are rare these days, and were more common in the days when the average diet was likely to be lacking in one respect or another. It is thought that these excessive cravings, called 'pica', were due to the body crying out for a desperately needed mineral such as iron, or for a deficient vitamin. Although this is now rare, most pregnant women certainly do still encounter changes in their likes and dislikes as far as food goes. These are not real cravings, however, just preferences. Try not to use this as an excuse to eat more sweet, sugary things, or more fattening items. My mother found she was strangely attracted to sour, unripe apples when pregnant, a craving that returned to her during the menopause; not just cooking apple sourness, but real acid, under-ripe, bitter sourness from the windfall apples which are normally discarded as inedible. This was fair enough in September, leading up to the birth of one of her children in October, but it was a bit more difficult to organize in May and June, when my own arrival was expected, and she had to make do with pickles instead! My husband's mother confessed to an abnormal, constant desire for raw, white cabbage, and during one pregnancy always carried a bag of chopped raw cabbage wherever she went, even on the bus, to munch when she got the uncontrollable urge. As well as acquiring a liking for certain foods you may not normally eat, you will probably also find that you come to dislike some foods which you normally enjoy. Luckily, pregnancy often brings with it a sudden distaste for smoking cigarettes, or drinking alcohol, both of which can be dangerous to the foetus. If you find that this happens to you, use the situation to your advantage and give up smoking for good. It will leave you and your baby healthier, and wealthier too. Encourage a smoking partner to do likewise. Smoking, even 'passive' smoking, is very, very bad for your baby. (For the effects of smoking on the foetus, see pp. 60–62.)

Haemorrhoids

Haemorrhoids, or piles, are painful varicose veins in and near the anus. They are caused by excessive pressure, for example from straining too hard to pass faecal matter when suffering from constipation, or from the pressure of the baby's head in the pelvic area very late on in pregnancy. Anyone who suffers from piles is likely to find that the problem recurs with subsequent pregnancies. It is more likely to occur in twin pregnancies. In order to help prevent piles, first prevent constipation (see p. 130). Follow a fibre-rich diet, and eat plenty of raw vegetables and fresh fruit, leaving the skins on. If piles become very troublesome or sore, consult your doctor; he may prescribe pain-relieving creams until your baby is born. After the birth, the piles will probably disappear of their own accord as the pressure is relieved.

Heartburn

This is a common symptom from mid pregnancy onwards, and it is an unpleasant side effect of having a baby inside you pushing up against your stomach as it takes up all the available space to grow. The sensation of heartburn is caused by small amounts of the contents of your stomach re-entering your oesophagus through the stomach valve at the top. This happens because of the pressure from the baby and also because, as with the digestive tract at the other end, the muscles of the digestive system relax during pregnancy because of increased hormone levels. If you regurgitate in this way several times in a row the oesophagus becomes sore and inflamed, making the symptoms worse than ever. The symptoms often become worse at night when you lie down, because the contents of your stomach can more easily move back up again. The best thing to do is to take lots of very small meals during the day, and to avoid eating large quantities of food in one go. This means that your stomach only ever has a small portion of food in it, but at the same time is never left completely empty, or made too full. Sometimes a glass of milk, sipped slowly, helps to relieve the 'burning' sensation. It is also a good idea to stay propped upright during the night if it gets very bad. A few extra pillows or cushions will help you to stay more upright while you sleep, and it is actually very comfortable to sleep in a sitting position. Avoid eating spicy or vinegary foods and drinking alcohol. Don't ever let your stomach become really empty, as this is when the acid in your stomach increases. Try not to bend over unnecessarily, as lowering your head below your chest will make heartburn more likely. Bend from the knees, not from the waist. Heartburn is more likely to occur in twin pregnancies because of the extra bulk and pressure that two babies obviously cause.

High blood pressure

At the beginning of pregnancy, up to about the twelfth or fourteenth week, the blood pressure is actually lower than normal (see 'Fainting and dizziness', p. 133). After this time the blood pressure usually returns to its normal level, and should remain at or slightly above this level until labour begins. Every time you visit your antenatal clinic your blood pressure will be measured, because rising blood pressure could herald the beginnings of certain complications of pregnancy, such as toxaemia, which need special attention and care. If you gain too much weight this will also raise your blood pressure, so try to keep your weight gain at a reasonable level. Any physical movement such as running or jumping will temporarily raise your blood pressure, but it should return to normal after a short period of rest. You will be more prone to high blood pressure if you are the sort of person who tends to be nervous, highly strung or easily agitated, or if you have a particularly stressful lifestyle. If this is the case, do your best to rest when you start to feel yourself becoming tensed up, and try to avoid any unnecessary nerve-racking activities such as watching the late-night horror movie on television.

Insomnia

Insomnia, or sleeplessness, is usually most troublesome during the last few weeks of pregnancy, when the baby is large and often lies awkwardly inside you. Some women find that the baby seems to kick and jump about more during the night, and is correspondingly less active during the day. This may be simply because you notice the kicking more when you lie down and keep still in bed, or because the baby is soothed in the daytime by the swaying movements of your body as you move around, or is subdued by the sound of your voice. Whatever the reason, a kicking, very mobile baby inside your tummy can be disturbing when you are trying to rest. The baby's movements become most noticeable after the thirtieth week of pregnancy, because his muscles are growing and becoming stronger and he still has enough space inside you to move around a lot. At the end of pregnancy the movements often become less noticeable and slow down, because the baby fills up all the available space inside you and has less room for manoeuvre.

Stress and worry can also cause insomnia, and if you are at all worried about any aspect of your pregnancy or are concerned about the approaching birth, talk to your partner, doctor or midwife, or all three, and discuss your worries with them. Most likely, the worries will disappear once you have voiced them.

You may find that although you are well able to get to sleep when you first retire to bed, you are woken up a few hours later by the baby kicking you, or by the desire to pass water, and cannot get back to sleep afterwards. If you find you are having to get up in the night to go to the lavatory, try not to drink any liquids after about 9 or 10 at night. This way you will have a better chance of getting through the night without being disturbed by the necessity to urinate. Try not to lie there worrying about not being able to get back to sleep, as this can become a vicious circle which can be difficult to break. Instead, try doing a few relaxing exercises, breathing exercises or yoga (there are special yoga exercises for pregnancy). Recite a favourite poem in your head, or say a prayer. Try not to drink any coffee during the day, as it is a mild stimulant which can keep you awake. Drink weak tea, fruit juices or herb teas instead. Camomile tea is said to have an especially soporific effect if taken last thing at night, or you could try a hot, milky drink. Before you retire, try consciously to relax and unwind for half an hour or so. Many pregnant women have a doze after lunch or during the afternoon – if you can't sleep at night, stop having that daytime nap and just sit quietly reading or listening to the radio with your feet up for half an hour or so instead. Then you may be able to get your full quota of sleep during the night. Please don't take any sleeping pills unless they are specifically prescribed for you during your pregnancy by your doctor, and make sure he knows you are pregnant before you ask for any. Don't use up any old sleeping pills you may have left over from before your pregnancy, as they could be dangerous to your baby. There are safe sleeping pills to take during pregnancy, but try to do without them if possible.

Nausea and morning sickness

Nausea: The feeling of sickness, without actually being sick, is called nausea. This is an extremely common symptom during the first three months of pregnancy, and is often one of the first real signs after a missed period to indicate that you may have conceived. The majority of pregnant women suffer from nausea even if they are never physically sick. In many cases this nausea occurs in the early morning on rising, although it can also happen later on in the day or in the evening. It is often made worse by cooking smells, or cigarette smoke, or even the fragrance of some perfumes. You may find you are more prone to travel sickness at this time too. Nausea during pregnancy is thought to be provoked by increased levels of hormones in the blood, particularly the hormone progesterone. In most cases the symptoms are at their most extreme around the tenth week of pregnancy, after which they start to get less severe again, usually disappearing completely by about the fourteenth week.

Morning sickness: While some women only *feel* sick, others are actually physically sick as the symptoms of nausea increase. Some women find they are more prone to retching first thing in the morning and before meals, when their stomachs are empty of food. Others suffer most after meals and cannot keep any food down for very long. If your sickness continues at a high level, you could find yourself starting to lose weight and feeling extremely weak and worn out. Don't worry about losing a little weight, but if you lose more than half a stone you should consult your doctor. Sickness saps your energy, and prolonged sickness can be extremely demoralizing and exhausting. However, about one in three women never suffer from any form of nausea or sickness at all during pregnancy.

Treatment is the same for both nausea and morning sickness, and there is a lot you can do to help yourself before you rush off to the doctor looking for medicinal relief. Remember the thalidomide tragedy, and do your best to prevent sickness rather than seek a cure for it. First of all, take everything very slowly. Don't leap out of bed first thing in the morning and start rushing about – slow down the pace of life and take things in your stride. Put a glass of water and a dry biscuit or a piece of bread beside your bed at night. When you wake up in the morning, slowly sip the water and nibble the biscuit or bread *before* you get out of bed, then lie still for ten minutes or so before you stand up. Many women find that this is enough to stop nausea altogether, and that if they can prevent the first attack in the morning they continue to feel well for the rest of the day. As the day progresses, make sure you get enough rest and continue to take things at a gentle, leisurely pace if you can. Take several short breaks throughout the day and rest quietly. Lie down, or doze, or sit in a comfortable chair, or sit cross-legged – do whatever makes you feel most comfortable.

Take care with your diet too. You may find the times and sizes of meals significant. Try eating six or seven small snacks throughout the day, instead of three conventional larger meals with long spaces in between. Try to eat a nutritious, varied diet with plenty of fresh fruit and vegetables. Don't eat fried or highly spiced foods, and keep away from alcohol. If you can't face eating much at all, consider taking a vitamin and mineral supplement. Vitamin B6 is thought to be very important for nausea, and the need for this vitamin does increase during pregnancy. Sometimes women may suffer from a deficiency of Vitamin B6 if they have been taking the contraceptive pill for a long time before trying to become pregnant. Try to get some fresh air every day – just a few minutes outside or a gentle walk will suffice. Wear loose clothes too; don't wear anything that will restrict you around the stomach, and discard any clothes that are too tight around the bust and tummy.

If all this fails and you are still suffering and being unbearably sick, ask your doctor for help. There are some safe drugs to take for pregnancy sickness, but please make sure you use them only as a last resort, if you just can't carry on normal life without some medicinal help. Before you take any pills, do your best to tackle the problem yourself.

Oedema

Oedema simply means swelling, and pregnancy can bring with it swelling of the feet, ankles, fingers, hands and face and can cause some puffiness all over the body. A certain amount of swelling is normal during pregnancy, due to the extra retention of water in the body caused by the pregnancy hormones, and can account for an increase in weight of around half a stone. This sort of swelling is usually most noticeable during the latter half of pregnancy, but oedema can occur at any time for other reasons. Swelling in the body can be caused in hot weather by overheating and by ill-fitting, over-tight shoes, but this usually disappears at night when it becomes cooler again. Severe swelling of the ankles, feet and hands which does not go away at night could be a symptom of the onset of toxaemia, and should be reported to your doctor. The intake of salt encourages the retention of water, so cut down on salt in your cooking as a preventive measure. Also avoid standing around for long periods of time without rest – sit down whenever you have the chance, and if possible put your feet up on a stool.

Palpitations

It sometimes happens in pregnancy that you can feel the beating of your heart more acutely than at other times, and sometimes you can 'hear' it beating inside you too. Occasionally you may also feel as if your heart misses a beat, or beats irregularly, or beats very fast, and all these sensations are called palpitations. This is perfectly normal, so don't worry about it at all. Your heart has a lot of extra work to do while you are pregnant, and needs to pump enough blood around your body to supply both you and your baby with the oxygen and the nutrients you need. Your blood supply increases in volume by around 40 per cent to keep up with the demand, so it is not really surprising if you notice a slight difference occasionally in the way your heartbeat sounds. To cope with the extra volume of blood needed by the body, the heart actually enlarges so that it is more powerful. This enables it to pump through the extra blood without speeding up the rate of the heartbeat (except for the occasional flutter). Palpitations are nothing to worry about. You will probably notice the sensation more when you undertake any physical activity, such as climbing the stairs, or even walking.

Passing water

At the beginning of pregnancy your desire to pass water often increases, so that you may need to visit the toilet far more frequently than usual. You may find you have to get up in the night to relieve yourself too. This is quite normal, and there is nothing much you can do about it except perhaps to limit your intake of liquid during the evening in the hope that you will be able to last through the night without having to get out of bed. Later on in pregnancy, about three-quarters of the way through, the need to pass urine more frequently may occur again. At this stage of pregnancy it is caused by the sheer bulk of the baby inside you, which presses down on your bladder and restricts the space normally reserved for the storage of urine. Again, there is nothing much you can do about it, so until the baby is born you will just have to get used to the routine of rising in the night to urinate.

Tiredness

Tiredness and extra sleepiness are normal signs of pregnancy, especially in the early months, and should be regarded as a signal to slow down. You do need more rest during pregnancy, so take it easy and try not to overdo things at this stage. You will probably need around ten hours sleep every night. Some women achieve this by sleeping for a couple of hours in the afternoon, but if you can't manage this because of work or other children to look after, do your best to get to bed early. Very often the extra tiredness disappears after about three months, but you should still try to get plenty of rest. Tiredness often returns during the last third of pregnancy, due to the extra weight you are carrying around with you and the extra demands the growing baby makes on your body. You just won't be able to move around so freely at this stage, so try not to arrange anything strenuous, such as moving house, during the latter half of your pregnancy. Extra rest during the last few weeks is essential for another reason too – you will soon be getting up two or three times a night to deal with night feeds, and you will need to have a good reserve of energy to be able to cope well at this time.

Toxaemia

This condition is also known as pre-eclampsia, and needs careful watching and plenty of rest in order to prevent it getting any worse and turning into eclampsia, which is a more severe form of the same thing. Toxaemia usually occurs only during the last few weeks of pregnancy, and is diagnosed by three distinctive symptoms. Any of these symptoms appearing by itself does not mean you have toxaemia – it is only when they all appear together that the condition is diagnosed. The first symptom is high blood pressure. Blood pressure is measured and recorded by two figures, one above the other, for example 120/70. Blood pressure is considered to be high when the bottom figure reaches 90 or more, i.e. 120/90. (A bottom figure of 60 or 70 is normal.) The second sign of toxaemia is oedema in the body, or swelling of the hands, feet, ankles and face. A certain amount of swelling is normal in pregnancy, but a trained doctor or nurse will be able to distinguish between this and the sort of swelling that is dangerous. The third sign of toxaemia is protein in the urine, and this is one of the reasons why your urine is tested every time you visit the antenatal clinic. These three symptoms are usually accompanied by an excessive weight gain, above the level which is normally expected at this stage of pregnancy. Once the condition is diagnosed the treatment is usually complete bed rest in hospital with careful monitoring of the symptoms, and this is usually enough to prevent it becoming any worse.

Vaginal discharge

Most women of childbearing age have a whitish vaginal discharge in their non-pregnant state. In pregnancy you can expect this to increase, because the glands at the neck of the cervix increase their output at this time. In every other respect the discharge should be exactly the same as before – there should just be more of it. If you notice a change in the colour from white to yellow or green, if it becomes itchy or irritating, or if it becomes very much thicker and smells unpleasant, you could be suffering from a minor infection. If you notice any or all of these signs, consult your doctor. This sort of infection is quite harmless and easy to treat with creams or pessaries. If you notice any blood in the discharge, however little, consult your doctor immediately. Vaginal bleeding does not necessarily mean danger, but it should be checked as soon as possible in order to find out the cause.

Varicose veins

Varicose veins can appear at any time during pregnancy but they are most likely to be bothersome during the second half. They occur when the veins become distended due to pressure. Once noticed, they can be prevented from developing by making sure you don't stand around for long periods of time without moving, and by remembering not to cross your legs when you are sitting down, as this reduces the circulation. It also helps if you can put your feet up on a stool or another chair whenever you sit down, so that the pressure in your legs is relieved. A small amount of exercise is also helpful, as this helps to get the circulation going. Take care not to restrict the blood flow in your legs – discard any stockings or over-the-knee socks that are tight around the top, and never use garters to hold up loose ones. However, you can wear support tights, and these will also be helpful in preventing the varicose veins from becoming worse.

7

Involving Your Man

These days, the father's supportive role throughout pregnancy and during birth is accepted as desirable and normal. Most fathers want to be involved right from the start, to be part of the active development of their family. This is a great help to any mother-to-be, as it is most important during your pregnancy to have close contact and support from a partner who can give you reassurance about the coming birth and who can share in as much of the process of pregnancy and birth as possible. For most of you, your husband will fit the bill perfectly (or your lover, if you don't happen to be married to him), but for others this may not be possible. Whatever your situation, try to involve somebody else in your pregnancy to give you support; it doesn't have to be a husband, it can be another woman if you prefer. You may be a single parent-to-be, not living with the father of your child, or your husband may be away from home a lot of the time, for example in the armed forces, and you may need someone else as your helper. A sister or brother would do very well, or a close friend, preferably one who lives very near by. You could also consider asking your mother, or another pregnant woman in a similar position to yourself, or a neighbour. It doesn't matter who it is, as long as you have somebody you can talk to about the events of pregnancy and with whom you can discuss any worries, problems, fears, desires and hopes. Throughout this chapter I shall refer to this helper as your 'man', 'husband' or 'partner', as this is the most usual arrangement, but please take it as understood that this includes anyone else who may be helping you.

Try to involve your man in all your preconception routines if possible, that is, if you have time to contemplate preconception care and put it into practice before conceiving. Ideally, you and your man should start sharing the responsibilities of parenthood even before your baby is conceived, as discussed in Chapters 3 and 4. After all, the male sperm is just as important and vital to conception as the female egg. Neither of you can become a parent without the help of the other, and it is vital for both sperm and egg to be as healthy as possible before joining to form a new being. In the months leading up to a planned conception you can *both* take measures to make yourselves as healthy as possible. For instance, if you smoke, you can give up cigarettes together. You are more likely to succeed if you have each other for moral support, to help get through the inevitable periods of weakness. You can both concentrate on changing your diet, so that you are eating the sort of body-building foods needed to be at the peak of health. You can both do without alcohol for a while; it will be much easier for you not to succumb to drink if your husband is not sitting in the corner drinking beer. Both of you can abstain from drug-taking. If you have been on the pill for any length of time before deciding to start (or to continue) your family, your body will need time to get back to normal – perhaps your husband can take the initiative for contraception for a change by using the sheath. Now is also the time for both of you to discuss with your doctor any long-term medical problems, such as diabetes, epilepsy or haemophilia, which are known to exist in either family. Some diseases are hereditary, so before you conceive, find out together if your future children are at risk so that you can make well-informed decisions about the implications of having a family. Your husband should also think about his place of work – is he exposed to any dangerous chemicals that might affect his fertility or the health of his sperm? You can both make an effort, together, to get some regular exercise too. It needn't be anything violent, just a gentle walk each day will be better than nothing. Whatever you do, it's much more fun to do it together. Eating a healthy diet is most definitely a joint endeavour – it's no good you eating salads and fruit if he demands crisps and jam doughnuts. You need help and sympathetic encouragement in order to better your diet. Work out what you are aiming to do together, and then put the plan into action. Encourage your man to read this book, especially the two chapters (3 and 4) concerned with preconception care and preconception diet, as these two things are as important for him to be aware of as they are for you. These are the first steps a man can make towards being a caring parent and husband.

Conceiving your baby, together

Once you decide the time has come to start trying to conceive, your husband can continue to help in other ways. You are at your most fertile at a certain time each month, and if you work out the dates as accurately as you can, you will know when to make love in order to give yourself the best chance of conceiving. Remember to double check the dates just in case you've made a mistake. You may not conceive straight away, and it may take several months, but if you know when your fertile days are you will have a better chance of succeeding quickly. A woman usually has a period every 28 days, but the time between periods can be longer or shorter than this depending on the individual. If your periods are always the same number of days apart, you will be able to work out your most fertile days quite accurately. If your periods are not regular, you can still get fairly close to knowing your fertile time, perhaps being able to pinpoint the week in which your most fertile day is likely to fall.

To work out a woman's most fertile time, let's take a 28-day menstrual cycle as a typical example. The first day of bleeding when a period starts is called Day 1. The bleeding usually continues for 4 or 5 days, perhaps ending on Day 5. Ovulation usually happens 14 days *before* the next period is due, and in a 28-day cycle this will be 14–15 days after the first day of the last period. Ovulation is the name given to the time when an egg is released from the ovary and moves down to the womb ready for fertilization, so the most fertile day is when ovulation takes place. If intercourse takes place once the egg has been released from the ovary, pregnancy is very likely.

However, the most fertile day will differ for a woman whose menstrual cycle is longer or shorter than 28 days. For instance, for a woman whose normal, regular cycle is 32 days, the most fertile day will be Day 18 (still 14 days *before* the next period is due). Sperm have the ability to live inside the womb and around the fallopian tubes for two or three days, so it follows that if you concentrate your love-making activities just before, as well as on, the actual most fertile day, you are quite likely to succeed in conceiving a baby.

If your menstrual cycle is completely irregular, you will need to work out an 'average' fertile time. For example, if the shortest ever gap between periods is 26 days and the longest ever gap is 35 days, you can link the two most probable fertile days (one from each length of cycle), and the time between those two days will be your *probable* most fertile time – in this particular case, it will last 14 days. This is shown in Fig. 14 (iii). Your actual most fertile day each month will lie somewhere inside those two weeks, and if you concentrate on having intercourse around the middle of that time every month, you should succeed in conceiving within a few months. If you have been unsuccessfully trying for a baby for more than a year, consult your doctor for expert advice.

If you suspect you have conceived, a proper pregnancy test will confirm your hopes. The usual earliest time for a test is 42 days (6 weeks) after the first day of your last period, or when your next period is about 2 weeks overdue. You need to wait this long to be sure of getting an accurate result. You can buy a pregnancy testing kit at any chemist's shop if you would like to do the test yourself, at home with your husband, or you can make arrangements to visit your doctor or clinic together. You will be asked to take an early morning sample of urine with you, as the early morning is the time when the hormone which indicates pregnancy is most likely to be present in sufficient quantities to be identified. When you get the result of the test it is nice to have someone else

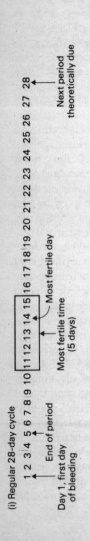

(i) Regular 28-day cycle

1 2 3 4 5 6 7 8 9 10 11 12 13 14 15 16 17 18 19 20 21 22 23 24 25 26 27 28

Day 1, first day of bleeding

End of period

Most fertile time (5 days)

Most fertile day

Next period theoretically due

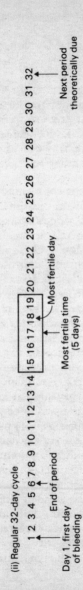

(ii) Regular 32-day cycle

1 2 3 4 5 6 7 8 9 10 11 12 13 14 15 16 17 18 19 20 21 22 23 24 25 26 27 28 29 30 31 32

Day 1, first day of bleeding

End of period

Most fertile time (5 days)

Most fertile day

Next period theoretically due

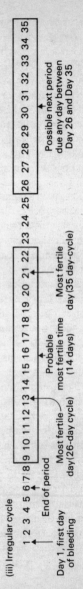

(iii) Irregular cycle

1 2 3 4 5 6 7 8 9 10 11 12 13 14 15 16 17 18 19 20 21 22 23 24 25 26 27 28 29 30 31 32 33 34 35

Day 1, first day of bleeding

End of period

Most fertile day (26-day cycle)

Probable most fertile time (14 days)

Most fertile day (35 day-cycle)

Possible next period due any day between Day 26 and Day 35

Fig. 14. Calculating your most fertile day.

with you to celebrate, or to commiserate if you find you are not pregnant after all.

Sharing and caring, right from the start

Once your baby is conceived, your man can share in much of the inevitable miscellany of events that occur during pregnancy, so that he feels part of the event and not an outsider. Of course he can't share in the feelings of morning sickness or heartburn (although it has been known for expectant fathers to come out in sympathy with their wives and suffer similar symptoms occasionally), but he can play an important part in the development of your future family by talking over and discussing with you the way you both feel now that the baby is a reality. It is good for you to talk things over together, because you are both bound to have a few lingering worries and nagging doubts about the next few months, especially if this is your first child. It is particularly important for your man to discuss the events of pregnancy and explore how it affects you, because it may be difficult otherwise for him to accept that the baby really exists at first. After all, he can't feel the symptoms of pregnancy, so he may not be able to visualize the baby as a real person. He can't see it yet, and he won't be able to feel it like you will when it grows big enough to start kicking inside. So read the pregnancy books together, and keep talking about the way in which your lives are changing. Keep your man informed about little details as well as the larger, more obvious signs. Be prepared to listen to his problems and fears as well as voicing your own. Share as many of the day-to-day occurrences and milestones of pregnancy as possible. If your man can accompany you to antenatal classes, so much the better. There you will both be able to learn about the events of labour and how to cope with contractions. The physiological side of pregnancy and birth will be explained, and it will bring home the truth of the matter – that the baby is already an important part of both of your lives.

The first physical sign of the baby that your man will be

able to appreciate is probably the beating of its heart. The baby's heart starts beating at the age of about seven weeks, but it will be quite a lot longer before anyone will actually be able to hear it with a stethoscope. Every time you visit the antenatal clinic, your doctor or midwife will regularly listen to your baby's heartbeat with a foetal stethoscope (like an old-fashioned hearing trumpet) placed over your tummy. Once you have been told that the heartbeat is audible, your man can try listening for it himself at home. He can try placing any hollow tube over your tummy, putting his ear to the other end to listen. (Try the inner cardboard tube from a kitchen roll or toilet roll.) It may take a few attempts before he can appreciate which noise inside you corresponds to what – digestion can be a noisy business, and he also needs to be able to distinguish your own heartbeat from the baby's. Remind him that the baby's heartbeat should sound very much faster than yours.

The reality of the baby will become still clearer to your man as your figure starts to change. By the time you are about 3½–4 months pregnant you will no longer be able to disguise the bump and the visual message will sink in, especially when he sees you without clothes, in the bath, or cuddled up in bed, where he can feel the curves as well as see them. Don't forget to tell him when you first feel the baby kick. This is another important milestone which helps to make the baby more real for the father. One day when it is particularly active, place his hand on your tummy so that he can feel it for himself. Sometimes the baby may kick quite violently, although it won't hurt you – it is lovely for your man to be able to feel it too, and he may be surprised by the strength of the baby's limbs.

Reassurance

Reassurance from each other is a very important need which both mother-to-be and father-to-be have during pregnancy. You both need to be assured and reminded that your fears and worries about pregnancy and birth, whatever they may be, are surmountable as long as you work together as a team. To begin with, once you find out for sure that you are pregnant you will both need reassurance of love. This is not as ridiculous or as obvious as it may sound. Pregnancy may have been the one thing you have both been wanting for months and months, but now that it has become a reality things may look different, even seeming like a threat to your husband. How can this be? Take a little time to think about it. You may both have had romantic dreams and fantasies about pregnancy and labour, and the reality of morning sickness, backaches and possible loss of libido may seem very different from what you had anticipated. You will need reassurance that you are still loved by your husband, and in the same way he needs reassurance that you still love him. You are both facing huge changes in your lives, especially with a first baby (and only slightly less so with subsequent children). Your consciousness is rapidly expanding and widening to include another person in your most immediate, personal life. Your husband may feel pushed out in the cold. Your body is changing too, growing larger and larger, and you both need one small but important stable foothold in the midst of all the changes – remember that love does not change, that love continues throughout all life, for better, for worse, for richer, for poorer, in sickness, in health and in pregnancy.

How your man can help you

For yourself, you will need encouragement and sympathy in a variety of ways during your pregnancy. You will need to be told that you are still attractive to your man, even while you are vastly expanding in all directions. It will help you a lot if your man can tell you that you are still both visually and sexually attractive to him, especially when you are feeling low, and a bit lumpy, like a sack of potatoes. (You *will* sometimes feel that way.) It will be a great help if your husband can show some sympathy for your symptoms of pregnancy too, as loving sympathy is better than any drug when you are feeling lousy. Compassion and commiseration are the best possible medicines at this time. An appreciation of your possibly volatile emotional state will also help. You may feel like exploding into various extremes of emotions for no apparent reason at all, perhaps giggling like a schoolgirl one moment and in floods of tears the next. It will be very helpful to you if you can rely upon your husband to realize that this is all due to hormones, and to expect the odd bit of unreasonable behaviour occasionally. It does not indicate emotional instability – it is just a temporary state of affairs. Your husband can help you by not rising to the bait if you suddenly recklessly blame all your present difficulties on him. Try to let him know that it's nothing personal, it's just a phase of pregnancy. Don't expect him to understand all this automatically – it needs explaining – so ask him to read this book, and any others you have, and to take time to discuss your feelings and his own.

Try to avoid unnecessary stress in your lives. This means both of you trying hard not to argue over trifling irrelevancies, and asking your husband to be patient and to talk things through with you when tempers flare. Talk any real differences of opinion through sensibly – the rest don't really matter. If you do end up fighting over anything, your husband would be very praiseworthy if he could cultivate his ability to forgive, and to remember that you are not quite yourself after all. Many marital fights are over trivialities, and leave the real, underlying, major difficulties unsolved. Neither husband nor wife needs to suffer in silence – talk to each other and discuss differences before they get out of proportion.

Your man can also help you to avoid stress by helping out with the housework now and then. At first he may think this sounds like unnecessary pampering, but early pregnancy can bring with it general lassitude, tiredness, irritability and an inability to cope with the normal run of events. Don't use it as an excuse to sit around all day, but do ask your man to help if you just can't manage. He could help with the cooking and washing up, and if he can't cook already, then now is the time to learn – accept burnt offerings with grace and hearty thanks for the effort. He could also help out with the weekly shopping, as it is not a good idea for you to carry heavy boxes and overloaded baskets now, but there is no need to shift all the responsibility to him—you can do it together. Remember not to *demand* help, but ask him nicely, just as you would expect in the reverse situation. During the last seven or eight weeks of pregnancy you won't be able to move around very much because of your size, so you'll need extra help especially then. If you already have some older children in the family, your man could help in ferrying them to and from school if you normally do it, and take them to the dentist's instead of you. Best of all, he needs to be able to do all these things without bearing a grudge, and without making scathing remarks about men doing women's work, as that will invalidate the helpfulness of any jobs he takes over.

How you can help your man

All this is really expecting quite a lot from your man, on top of any work responsibilities and other worries he may have. So be ready to give him reassurances too. Tell him he is still 'number one' in your life, and reassure him that the new baby is not going to displace him in your affections. Let him know that the baby is a joint interest, for both of you to share, and tell him that he is not being thrown out or pushed away from you, or removed from his place alongside you in his role as husband and lover. On the contrary, the baby should reinforce your togetherness and bind you more closely than ever. Men also sometimes need reassurance that they can be part of the act of birth, and that you will want and need them to be with you when the baby is born. Your man may be interested, but ignorant of any facts, so tell him how he will be able to help you throughout your labour (see p. 158). Let him know that you want him involved. Read the baby books together and encourage him to attend antenatal classes with you. Practise the breathing exercises together, so that he will know when you go wrong or when you lose your sense of rhythm during the actual labour, and will be able to put you back on the right track of breathing to counteract the strength of the contractions. Keep on making the baby a reality throughout your pregnancy. Let your man feel it kick and hear its heartbeat, and if an ultrasonic scan is done for any reason, perhaps to check the maturity and size of the baby to see if its size corresponds to your dates, take him along with you so that he can see the shape of the baby too.

Don't forget your role as your husband's lover. Some men are upset that their sex lives go downhill for a while during pregnancy, and feel shut out and distant as a result. Few women feel complete repulsion at the idea of sex during pregnancy – most loss of libido at this time is simply due to over-tiredness. It would be thoughtful of you to keep on taking care of your husband's sexual needs despite your lack of interest. If you really can't face intercourse itself, try to please your man in other ways. Don't ignore his sexual needs just because yours diminish – it will almost certainly cause emotional friction between you and lead to stress.

Lastly, don't suddenly demand extra money for a pram, pushchair, high chair, cot, etc. Work out your finances together, and be sympathetic and sensitive to the fact that your man will now feel extra financial responsibility for his growing family. Don't make him feel that he is failing you if he can't supply enough cash for everything at once, especially if you are giving up work to have the baby and are therefore losing some regular income. Work out your money supply together and plan accordingly. You still have plenty of time to save up for the larger items, and no doubt you will be showered with gifts and cast-offs from family and friends as the time of the baby's arrival gets nearer. If you are a bit short of cash, let your man know you are content with some second-hand baby equipment – this is often advertised in the local papers, and it's much cheaper to buy it that way. Let your husband talk about any fears and worries of his own that your pregnancy faces him with. Be sympathetic and loving, and he will respond in the same way. Your baby was conceived as a joint effort, so continue to do things together and share the joys and responsibilities of its birth and future development.

A few advance preparations

It is a good idea for you both to have a firm plan in your minds about what you will do when your labour begins. You should have all the details worked out beforehand, so that in the actual event you won't need to think too hard about what is happening and will just be able to follow the instructions already listed in your head, or on a piece of paper kept somewhere handy. After all, labour may start in the middle of the night, when are are not at your most scintillating or mentally alert. The excitement and/or apprehension may overwhelm you both, so you need to be confident that you will know exactly what to do when the time comes.

If you are planning to have your baby in hospital, your husband can help you by arranging all the transport details. If you have your own car, remind him to keep the petrol tank topped up as the expected date of delivery draws closer. (Don't be caught short – my first baby arrived three weeks early, so be prepared at least a month in advance!) If you don't have your own car you may be able to make arrangements with a relative, friend or neighbour to borrow one. If so, get used to driving it *before* the big day arrives. Failing that, you could plan to use a taxi. Check with the taxi firm in advance, don't just rely on using the telephone directory at the last minute – some firms may have gone out of business since the directory was printed, and others may not be prepared to transport a woman in labour. Ring around and ask first. Don't forget that in an emergency you can dial 999 for an ambulance, but *please* restrict the use of this service to a real emergency – don't expect to be able to use an ambulance as a free ferrying service. Whatever mode of transport you choose, try to have your suitcase packed in advance so that you can be ready to leave at a moment's notice. If you are not on the telephone, make arrangements with a neighbour to use theirs. If they offer to lend you a key so that you can still use their telephone if they are out when you need it, it is a good idea to leave the number of the hospital by their telephone in advance.

So, now you've got your transport, do you know where you are going? If your husband is going to be driving it is a good idea to plan a route to the hospital and make a test drive beforehand so that you know how long the journey takes. Some hospitals are very large and confusing, so find out which door you are supposed to use and where you can park nearby.

If you are planning to have your baby at home, your husband can help you to collect in advance all the bits and pieces you'll need during your labour, such as a large plastic sheet to protect the bed, various buckets and dishes for soiled dressings, etc. (your midwife will give you a list). Make it your husband's responsibility to telephone the midwife at the appropriate time, and make sure he knows the correct number and what name to ask for (write it down beside the telephone).

When labour starts

Once you are in labour and placed wherever you wish to be, at home or in hospital, your husband can continue to help you throughout the various stages. At first this will only amount to keeping you happy, by reading to you, talking, simply holding your hand, telling you jokes or walking around with you if that is what you want to do. Tell him in advance that you will not want to take this opportunity to discuss the state of the drains and sewerage at home, or to review the world football situation – you are the centre of attention at this point and should remain so, and whatever you require should be provided.

As soon as the contractions start to become more regular and stronger, your partner can help by timing the length of each contraction and by noting the length of time between them. As soon as each contraction is regularly lasting for a whole minute and there is not more than ten minutes between any two, you can assume that labour is progressing nicely and that the baby is definitely on its way. Your husband can continue his support by supplying you with anything else you require, such as extra pillows, paper hankies, books, etc. As the contractions become stronger you will need to stop whatever you are doing and concentrate on using your breathing exercises. Your husband can help by doing the breathing with you, to encourage you and to give you a pattern to copy when you lose your rhythm. He can also act as an interpreter between you and the staff. At times you may be incapable of protesting against certain procedures, such as episiotomy or the giving of pain-killing drugs, particularly at the height of a long, difficult contraction when you need all your energy and concentration to cope. During these times it is up to your husband to do the talking, and to let the doctors and nurses know what you do and do not desire. He can also be useful if you find you want to walk around, or squat, or take up any other position which seems comfortable. He can physically help you to get into a better position, and he can also make sure your wishes are not interfered with – after all, it is your baby and your body, and you ought to be able to give birth exactly how you want, provided you are not risking damage to the baby or yourself. You may also find that you would like your husband to massage your back, thighs, or tummy. A cool flannel for your face or a hot water bottle for your back can also be helpful. Your husband's role should be one of encouragement and sympathetic motivation throughout labour.

As soon as the baby is finally born and the cord is cut, your husband will be able to take the baby and bring it over to you, to look at together. Or if you prefer, you can ask for the baby to be placed straight on to your tummy as it is born, so that you have immediate physical contact. It is at this stage, or a short while afterwards, that many men rush off to telephone relatives and friends, or to join pals in the local pub for a celebration, or just to drop into a bed somewhere and sleep. However tired and exhausted a husband might feel, he can't possibly be as tired and exhausted as his wife, but for her the event is not yet over. For instance, you may have sustained a tear in the perineum during labour, or had a cut made (episiotomy) to ease the birth, which will need stitching up again. You may have to wait quite a long time for a doctor to arrive to perform this, perhaps with your legs in stirrups if you are badly torn and are still likely to bleed, and I have been told by many women and also know from my own experience that receiving the stitches can be the most painful part of the whole procedure. Ask for gas and air during stitching if you require it, and ask your husband to stay with you if you feel you need his company. You still need his support and love at this stage just as much as you did in labour. If he wants to feel that he has really done everything he can for you and looked after you perfectly, he will stay with you while you are stitched up, and wait until you are safely tucked up in bed again. Then he can go home to bed too, knowing that he has done everything within his power to make sure you are comfortable.

After the baby is born

Please explain to your husband that during the next few days you really want him to visit you *every* day, at least once, especially during the evening visiting hours. Life can sometimes seem terribly miserable if you are sitting all by yourself in a ward full of other people's visitors. It can make you feel really rejected and unloved if nobody comes to see you when all the other mothers have people visiting them. A prudent husband will arrange for a friend or relative to visit you instead, if there is a day when he just can't get to you himself.

Ideally, your husband's offer of help should not end with the delivery of the baby. When you arrive home you will still need help in learning to cope with your new baby routine. Contrary to popular belief, motherly love and the mothering instinct do not necessarily happen automatically. For many of us (and more often than not) it has to be learnt, through trial and error and long hours of practice. Your husband's help at this stage, physically, emotionally and spiritually, is still of vital importance. A father has to get to know his new child in the same way as its mother does, by spending time holding it, feeding it, and generally getting to know it day by day. Your man is perfectly capable of bathing the baby too, and if you are not breastfeeding he can give it its bottle and can also learn to make up the sterilized feeds to give you a break from the routine (even if only at weekends). There is no reason why he should not wash the cot sheets occasionally instead of you, and scrub the dirty nappies now and then, and lull the baby to sleep when it is fretful and crying. He can put the other children to bed and finish making the dinner now and again. In fact, a joint effort with everything is the best possible arrangement.

If your husband has a nine to five job he will still be able to help in the evenings. Probably the most exhausting part of parenthood during the first three months is dealing with night feeds, and it would be a bit unfair to expect your husband to join in there too if he has a daily job to go to, but if he is unemployed, as so many people are these days, there is no reason why he shouldn't also help at night. The more help he gives you at the beginning, the quicker you will be able to recover from the physical ordeal of childbirth. If, by his actions, he gives you extra time to rest, sleep and get your strength and energy back, you will be able to return to your normal, lively self more quickly.

Parenthood is a 24-hour a day, 7-day a week job, and the father's role can be as large or as small as each husband prefers. Sharing the work between you is the ideal arrangement, especially at the beginning, not just to give you time to recover physically and ease your work load but also so that your husband can share in the joyful parts of parenthood and have a chance to get to know his offspring more intimately. Babies change so fast and grow so quickly, and it would be a shame for any father to miss out on the earliest weeks by leaving everything to the mother. As you begin to recover and start to get your energy back, the load won't be so great and you will be able to balance out the work between you again, in whatever manner you choose. Perhaps your husband will concentrate on work again, in his traditional role as sole earner and provider, and you will concentrate on bringing up the family – or vice versa, if that is what you wish.

8

Physical Exercise and Preparation

Conditioning your body for birth

Birth itself is a time of great physical exertion, and it takes an enormous amount of energy and concentration to do it well. It is the 'grand finale' to pregnancy, the real crux of the whole matter, the reason your body has been preparing itself for all these months. The human body is quite capable of looking after itself during a normal pregnancy, and does all the right things automatically. The breasts swell and enlarge in readiness for feeding the baby, the pelvic girdle softens, and the cervix relaxes and lets go its tight hold as the birth approaches. The mother's blood supply increases to cater for the demands of the baby. All these things and many more occur quite naturally, often spurred into action by hormones. They are all involuntary actions of the body – you don't have to think about doing them, they happen all by themselves. Your body miraculously accommodates itself to cope, and it really is a marvellous feat of engineering with this built-in facility for change and growth.

Normal labour is also usually automatic, if left to its own devices. It starts of its own accord, and continues all by itself through one, two, and three stages, under normal circumstances, so you may ask why you should bother to make any effort to prepare yourself physically during pregnancy, or in readiness for the birth, if your body does it all anyway? The answer is quite simple. It is a great advantage to you to prepare yourself mentally and physically for birth. Nobody knows in advance just how the actual labour will turn out or progress; not everybody has a 'normal' labour, and however slight the variation, if you have mastered the simple art of breathing correctly and of using some breathing exercises to help you cope with the heavier contractions, you will have a better chance of keeping in control and of being aware of what is happening to you. There are also certain physical exercises that you can do regularly throughout pregnancy to strengthen your pelvic floor muscles, thereby decreasing the likelihood of sustaining a tear, or of needing an episiotomy. If you are going to use the breathing exercises to their full potential you will need to be able to *relax* properly too (not always easy in the middle of a strong contraction), and there are special relaxation techniques you can learn and practise to enhance the beneficial effects of the breathing exercises in labour. All these are different aspects of preparing your body to aid your labour, rather than to hinder it by ignorance. Details of each of these techniques are described later in this chapter. They should, ideally, be practised throughout the whole of pregnancy, so that they are second nature to you by the time you come to need them in labour, but it is never too late to start.

Conditioning your body for pregnancy

As well as exercising and learning relaxation in readiness for the birth of your baby, you can also use physical activity in a helpful way throughout the long months of pregnancy. For example, taking care to adopt the correct standing and sitting posture is very important during pregnancy (see pp. 116–21). Keep reminding yourself to check your posture in the mirror, and look at your reflection in shop windows as you go by – are you standing up straight or slouching along instead? Remember to use your stomach muscles instead of just letting them go: they are still there, and are still usable, even if they have become distended and rounded. Just because you can no longer hide your lump is no reason to just let it all flop and sag – keep using your stomach muscles to help to hold yourself erect. Look at pp. 117–18 to find out how you can check if your posture is correct, and how to alter it for the better if not.

Gentle exercise during pregnancy is all to the good. If you

are sitting down for most of the day because of the sort of work you do, it is a good idea for you to get outside for a walk now and again. Constant sitting and no exercise limits the circulation of blood – a gentle stroll will get it moving again, and will loosen up creaking, stiff muscles in the legs. If you are susceptible to varicose veins, regular, gentle exercise of this sort can help prevent them, as it encourages good circulation and the return of the blood from the legs to the heart and lungs, where the blood is re-oxygenated and sent around the body again. A sluggish return of blood to the heart and lungs can cause the veins in the legs to become varicose, and gentle walking encourages the blood to get moving again. Exercise also encourages deep breathing and makes you use your lungs, increasing the supply of oxygen to the rest of your body. Moderate exercise, for example gardening, cycling, yoga, dancing or swimming, is also very good during pregnancy if you feel up to it. (Remember to tell your instructor you are pregnant if you go to any exercise classes.) Some of the more active sports, such as tennis, golf or jogging, are also fine in early pregnancy so long as you have previously been used to taking part in such activities regularly. Obviously as you become larger and larger you will not feel like taking so much physical exercise, and you should always take care not to over-exercise so that you become exhausted. Most people can judge fairly accurately when their bodies have had adequate exercise, and can therefore avoid pushing themselves beyond their natural physical limits. No exercise should be taken to extreme in pregnancy – it is fine to jog a couple of miles slowly if you are used to doing so normally, but don't try running a marathon.

Some sports are too dangerous during pregnancy, and if continued could cause real problems, even resulting in miscarriage if taken to extremes. In horse riding, for example, there is always an element of risk involved, and it is just not worth chancing damaging yourself and perhaps your baby too, as could happen if you were thrown badly or awkwardly. Skills such as skiing or water-skiing can be dangerous, because you just don't have the same sense of balance or judgement during pregnancy and you could easily misjudge a situation which under normal circumstances would not be a problem for you. Just remember to know your limits – there are many other pleasant ways of taking exercise. Don't endanger yourself or your baby by overdoing things, and avoid sports such as motor racing or parachuting! It is mostly a matter of common sense, but if you are in doubt about whether any particular physical activity is safe during pregnancy, ask your doctor. Don't get overtired, and remember to rest adequately as well as ensuring that you get enough exercise.

Breathing exercises

Many women who are pregnant for the first time don't realize how helpful breathing exercises can be during labour, and therefore they don't bother to practise them enough. It is not easy to accurately imagine being in labour if you have only read about it and have not yet experienced it for yourself, and consequently the virtues of breathing exercises are often underestimated and undervalued. I would advise anyone who is pregnant to persevere with learning these, or similar breathing techniques, as they can be a real asset when the time comes for your baby to be born. Coupled with muscle relaxation techniques they will give you a much better chance of controlling the fiercer contractions, rather than giving in to feelings of inadequacy and letting the contractions rule you. Labour, as the name suggests, can sometimes be a very long, laborious affair, and if you are breathing well and are in command of the situation you will feel very much better. Using breathing exercises during labour gives you something to concentrate on, something definite to hold on to, something old and familiar when you are undergoing strange, new experiences. If you can succeed in concentrating on your breathing your mind won't have time to panic or wander off into fear-ridden fantasy. Instead, you will be actively involved in the birth of your baby – birth won't be something that just happens to you and is managed by others. You will be in control of your own body and able to rely on your own judgement to decide when and if you want any pain-killing drugs to help you along. The real aim of breathing well is to allow you to breathe comfortably and easily without tensing the muscles in your tummy. Any tension in the abdominal region covering the contracting uterus can cause the sensation of pain, so you need to be able to fill your lungs with air and empty them again without using the muscles around your tummy to do so. Normally, if you breathe in and out really deeply, you will be able to feel those tummy muscles over the womb moving too. At the very beginning of labour this poses no problem, as pain is seldom felt at this stage; indeed, deep breathing is positively helpful during early labour because it encourages you to relax into the natural rhythm of your labour at a time when you might feel over-excited and a bit edgy. As the contractions become longer, closer together and stronger, you will start to find that any pressure on top of your tummy increases the sensations of the contraction, making you feel more uncomfortable and causing extra pain. In this case, what is needed is shallower, faster breathing to ensure that you still get enough air without using those muscles around your stomach which are on top of your contracting uterus. There are three levels of breathing which can be used to advantage during this first stage of labour, when the cervix is dilating – full breathing, semi breathing and mini breathing. You can choose which level to use depending on the intensity of the contraction.

1. *Full breathing*. This can be done by breathing either in and out through your mouth, or in through your nose and out through your mouth. Full breathing uses all your lung capacity to breathe deeply and evenly. Breathe in and out to a slow, natural rhythm. Feel and become aware of the muscles you are using to breathe with and try to relax them. Let the contractions flow through you without tensing any muscles. Fill your lungs completely each time you breathe in, and take the same amount of time to empty your lungs as you do to fill

them. As you breathe out let all tensions go with the breath. Full breathing is useful in early labour, before the contractions become strong enough to disturb you. Use full breathing to relax you and keep your whole body limp, just concentrating on keeping calm and steady, to stop you getting too excited or jumpy. As your contractions become more intense and you feel that full breathing is not enough to keep you abreast and in control of your labour, move up to the next level.

2. *Semi breathing.* Semi breathing is faster and shallower than full breathing, so that your tummy muscles do not move so much. Use your mouth for breathing both in and out. Semi breathing should be about twice as fast as full breathing, and you need to fill your lungs only half as full with each breath, so the overall effect is very much shallower and quicker. Use semi breathing at the height of a contraction, as you need it, returning to full breathing whenever possible. (In other words, return to full breathing at the beginning and end of each contraction, and also use it between contractions.) You can use semi breathing for the peaks of contractions during most of the first stage of labour, but if the contractions keep getting stronger and you seem to be in danger of getting out of control, you can move up to the third level.

3. *Mini breathing.* Use only your mouth for mini breathing. Don't try using your nose. This is very fast and shallow indeed, a bit like panting, but more controlled. Keep your diaphragm as still as possible (but not at all rigid), and suck and push the air in and out of your mouth without gasping. You should use this type of breathing only at the very height of the strongest contractions, reverting to semi breathing as soon as possible and finally relaxing back into full breathing again as the contraction passes. In the same way, start off every contraction with full breathing, moving on up to semi and mini breathing as necessary. A contraction at the end of the first stage of labour should look something like Fig. 15.

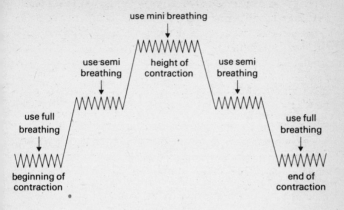

Fig. 15. A typical contraction at the end of the first stage of labour, showing how to use breathing exercises.

Breathing in the transitional stage

The transitional stage of labour is just what the name suggests, the time between the first stage of labour, when the contractions are still opening up the cervix, and the actual delivery of the baby. Between these two stages of labour there may be a short time when you have an overwhelming urge to push the baby out, but are told to hold back until the cervix has completely dilated and opened up. Then you must be able to prevent yourself from pushing for just a few moments longer, until the way is quite clear for the baby to descend. There are two techniques which will help you deal with this particularly trying stage – use one or both of them, whichever you find most effective at the time.

1. *Blowing hard.* This consists of a sharp expelling of the air in your lungs just when you feel the urge to push. A short, sharp 'BLOW', a bit like the sound you make after a lucky escape – 'phew!' Try to keep your muscles relaxed at the same time and to avoid gasping. Keep the rhythm steady.

BLOW – small breath in – BLOW – small breath in – BLOW – small breath in – BLOW. Keep this up during each contraction until the desire to push fades as the contraction diminishes in strength.

2. *The 'P' technique*. This is simply a repetition of the sound that the letter P makes: P-P-P-P-P-P-P-P-P-P-P. It should be executed at a very fast rate indeed, and should sound a bit like machine-gun fire. Keep it as rapid and loud as you can. Get your husband to help you with this one, and don't be afraid of making a fool of yourself! Ask him to do it with you, so that you have an example to follow.

Breathing for the birth itself

After the transitional stage, the birth itself will probably seem utter simplicity. All you have to do now is push, and the urge to push may be so great that you can just follow your own instincts and push the baby out without further ado. But it is useful to remember one particularly important point – as you push for all you are worth, remember to relax the birth outlet at the same time. It is not much good pushing and pushing from above if the entrance to your vagina is screwed up tight so that the head of the baby cannot easily pass through it. Sometimes the urge to push brings with it this desire to tense up all the muscles in the pelvic floor, so try to become aware of the sensations there and relax the opening as you push.

Take a few breaths of full breathing (see p. 167) as you feel the desire to push come upon you, and as the desire gets stronger hold your breath at the end of a deep breath in, when your lungs are completely filled with air. Now push hard, down and out, pushing the baby along the vagina steadily, out into the world. When you need more air, breathe in again and then hold your breath once more to push, repeating this until the desire to push starts fading. You may feel yourself going red in the face with the effort involved. Remember to keep the birth outlet open and loose.

Relaxation

You need to be able to relax all the muscles in your body if you are to use the breathing exercises to their full advantage. If your whole body is tensed up in pain, twisted and locked into a muscle-bound heap, you will not be able really to take charge of your labour. So it is useful to practise relaxation techniques during pregnancy, especially if you are a hyperactive type or if you are easily disturbed and unnerved by strange surroundings and new experiences. When labour begins, you are almost bound to feel excited, and probably nervous. You need to be able to use relaxation to settle yourself down again. Relax your mind and your body together, so that the sensations of your contractions can filter through you without you reacting with tenseness. If you can relax the necessary muscles, the contractions of labour will wash over you and flow naturally through you, and you will be able to let them do their work of dilating the cervix without blocking them with taut tummy muscles.

Relaxation is a matter of letting stress flow out and away from you, away from your body, away from your mind. Mental stress can cause your body to react physically by tensing up, as seen if you wring your hands in despair, or grit your teeth in a nerve-racking situation. This tensing up often happens when you know a situation is going to be difficult to handle, and often the expectation is worse than the fact. When you are lying down and relaxing into labour, you need to be able to lose the rigidity which normally holds your body erect when standing. It is not always easy to do this, and it can be difficult to let go completely, especially if you are expecting to feel pain, but it can be learned and practised. You need to be able to let fear go, to cooperate with your body in labour, to respect the magnitude of the event and not to fight against it. You should be able to surrender to the natural process of birth and not hinder it by blocking it with taut, intractable muscles and an unyielding, stiff body. Once you are in labour you can work on dissolving any feelings of fear or panic that remain. Think of your body as if it were made of rubber – it is stretchy, supple and elastic, it is springy, flexible and versatile, it was designed for birth so let it do its work without hindrance. Don't let your muscles fossilize into a rigid mass, soften them and let them go loose. Feel yourself becoming fluid and limp. Breathe deeply and evenly.

To practise relaxation

Lie down in a comfortable position with cushions and pillows supporting your head and upper back. Close your eyes and gradually, bit by bit, let go of any tension in the body. Start with your face. Let your eyes go heavy, then your nose and mouth. Breathe in through your nose and out through your mouth, connecting in your mind the breath out with a feeling of 'tension out'. Release any muscles still held by tension. Unclench your teeth, let your jaws loosen. Become aware of your scalp and brow – are they still tensed up? Let them go. Concentrate on your shoulders in the same way next, then your arms, hands and fingers, then your tummy and the muscles in your pelvic floor. Feel the weight of your body pressing against the floor. Imagine that you are stuck to the floor with glue, that you are fixed there in this blissful, relaxed state. Just relax completely, and imagine yourself actually sinking into the floorboards. Relax your legs, knees, feet and toes in the same way. Feel the power of gravity pulling your whole body down, down, into peaceful rest. When your whole body is as completely relaxed as possible, concentrate especially on the muscles in your tummy. These are the muscles you will particularly need to be able to relax during labour, so that they will not work against the pull of the uterus contracting beneath them. Tensed up stomach muscles on top of your contracting womb will not be helpful and may increase the amount of pain you feel. Imagine your womb contracting (like a very strong period pain), and then consciously let go of any tautness in the stomach muscles above. Imagine letting the contraction flow through you without resisting it physically. Help your womb to do its work by cooperating with your body and just relaxing into the process of labour.

Physical exercises

While you are pregnant you can do two kinds of physical exercises which will be beneficial to you. They are: (1) Physical exercises to keep your whole body fit and mobile in pregnancy, such as the general loosening up exercises to keep your limbs and muscles supple which are often done at ordinary keep fit classes. These may need to be modified to suit your present condition, but they will not differ drastically from a normal keep fit routine. (2) Physical exercises for the pelvic floor. These are designed specifically to strengthen the muscles surrounding the entrance to the vagina, and thereby to increase your awareness and control of these muscles, which have to stretch quite a lot as your baby is born.

General keep fit exercises

If you are used to doing a regular amount of keep fit exercises, pop mobility, yoga, aerobics or something similar once or twice a week, there is no reason why you should not continue to do so during pregnancy, at least during the early stages. Obviously extra care has to be taken to avoid overtaxing yourself, and you must also be careful not to take part in any exercise routines that are uncomfortable or that stretch the wrong muscles. As soon as your lump starts to get in the way of your normal routine you should adapt each exercise to keep it comfortable and easy, without strain.

If you have not previously been used to much exercise of any sort then it is probably wise just to continue as before. (Now is not the time to learn a new dance technique.) If, however, you are already a member of a keep fit class then let your instructor know that you are pregnant as soon as possible, and take his or her advice about slowing down your physical activities. You are obviously not going to attempt any back-flipped somersaults, for instance, but there is no reason why you should not continue to take part in a gentler routine. Best of all, start attending some proper antenatal classes, where you can safely learn how far you should go and find out what to avoid. A good guide is to stick to what is still comfortable for your body – you should never take part in any activity which exhausts you or causes you discomfort or pain. You may find that your body will automatically regulate your physical movements for you. You may feel much too tired to take part in anything at all (in which case don't push it), or your body may allow you to do a little though you find you tire much more quickly and easily than you used to. Let your body be your guide. Expect to do less, expect to feel tired sooner than before, and remember that there are some things you simply *cannot* do at the moment. Be aware of the need to slow down, and put the safety of your baby above all else.

Physical exercises for the pelvic floor

These involve any activity which uses and strengthens the muscles of your pelvic floor, or which increases your awareness of these muscles so that you can easily contract and release them at will. (This may not be as easy as it sounds.) These exercises have a dual purpose. In the first place the muscles around the vagina, the vaginal opening itself and the perineum need to be strong, supple, elastic and flexible, so that when your baby is born the perineum is less likely to tear or rip, and more likely to stretch adequately to let the baby through without necessitating stitching. This is a great advantage. To give birth without needing any stitches is a real joy and a really praiseworthy achievement – certainly something that is worth working for. Second, you should learn to release and relax these muscles at will, because as your baby is born you will need to *relax* the whole of the vaginal opening, at the same time pushing the baby out using other muscles above. So you need to be able to tense and push with some msucles, and at the same time be aware of and be able to relax others in the birth outlet. Some women can do this automatically, while others need to practise. The main problem is that pain, or more importantly the fear of pain, can cause these muscles to bind up tightly and be rigid without you realizing it. If this happens, then as you are pushing the baby downwards you will be pushing *against* your tightened pelvic floor – one set of muscles will be working against another set, and this will almost certainly result in a tear of the perineum which will need stitching up again afterwards. You won't know in advance, if this is your first baby, how you will react in labour, so it's just as well to practise anyway.

The best way to practise the use of these muscles is simply to use them regularly, practising the art of tensing them and then letting them go lax again, and training yourself to be able to contract and then relax them at will. You can work up to doing this regularly, ten to twenty times a day, and this should be enough to make your pelvic floor muscles strong and flexible. There are several ways in which you can exercise these muscles, and I have described five below. Either choose one which suits you best and practise it once or twice a day, or choose a different exercise each day.

1. *Squatting*. Stand up straight, feet apart, and slowly lower your body down until you are in a squatting position. You should be able to feel the muscles of your pelvic floor contracting as you lower your body down. Try relaxing your pelvic muscles in the squatting position. Then tense them again. Slowly stand up again.

2. *Tampon*. Imagine that inside your vagina you have a tampon which is falling out, and try to hold it in using only the vaginal muscles. Then relax. Now imagine pushing it right out with your vagina. Relax again. Now try pulling it back in again, just using those muscles in the pelvic floor. Become aware of the muscles you are using.

3. *Urgency to urinate*. Imagine that you are desperate to reach a lavatory to urinate, and have to wait in a queue.

Imagine having to hold back the flow of urine till you find an available toilet. Try the same exercise, this time imagining you are holding back faecal matter instead. Notice that you use slightly different muscles for this type of control. Although there are two different sets of muscles, one for each area, they are nevertheless connected and you cannot contract one without affecting the other slightly.

4. *Stopping the flow*. Do this one when you are sitting on the lavatory to urinate. Let a little urine out and then stop the flow again. Repeat until the bladder is empty. If you can easily stop the flow of urine at will in this way, you should not have much trouble in releasing these muscles for birth too.

5. *Sexual activity*. One of the nicest things about sex in pregnancy is that it is also good for your pelvic floor muscles. As the vagina grips the penis during lovemaking, your pelvic floor muscles are contracting. Practise contracting and relaxing them during intercourse – you and your partner may both find this interestingly erotic, as well as it being a good exercise to strengthen your pelvic floor.

Athletics in the womb

Your baby needs exercise too! As you are preparing yourself physically for birth, the baby itself will be doing the same, by kicking and jumping and squirming about inside you so that its own muscles are frequently used and thereby strengthened, ready for life in the outside world. These movements are usually not felt by the mother until around the nineteenth or twentieth week of pregnancy with a first baby, and a little earlier with subsequent babies. The baby actually starts moving about long before this, but the movements are not sufficiently strong to be felt before this stage. Mothers-to-be often complain that as soon as they lie down at night to sleep, the previously quiet baby starts jumping around inside them. This is probably because as they move around during the day they are thinking of other matters and simply don't notice much of the gentler movement, and also because the baby may like the swaying movements of its mother's body as she walks about and may be quietened by this kind of motion. Certainly, after birth, this kind of swaying motion in the arms of its mother lulls a baby to sleep.

9

Sex in Pregnancy

The unique human being

The human female is a special case in the world of animal biology and psychology, because she is one of the very few mammals in the world (perhaps the only one) which allows sex to continue after conception and throughout pregnancy. The precise reasons for this are still being debated, but most probably it is simply because female humans enjoy sex as much as their partners do, and wives are as loath to give it up as their husbands are. Many couples see continued intimacy throughout pregnancy as part of the blossoming of the pregnancy itself, especially where the baby was planned in advance and is a very much wanted addition to the family. After all, a baby is conceived during a session of lovemaking which is usually a tender and sensitive expression of love between two people, and there is no reason why this caring situation should not continue throughout pregnancy for as long as is comfortable and desirable for both partners. Each couple is different, and each prospective father and each mother-to-be react in varying, individual ways to the news of a pregnancy. There is no doubt that pregnancy *changes* the sexual side of our lives, and that we have to accommodate ourselves to these changes and learn to plan around the difficulties, but few couples would give up sex altogether just because there is a baby on the way. There are some (but only a few) special circumstances in which sex is undesirable, and where doctors will advise couples to refrain from sexual relationships, if only for a short time (see p. 186), but in most normal cases doctors encourage the continuation of a loving relationship between husband and wife, for the benefit of all.

Taking care of your man

Pregnancy can occasionally cause some psychological problems, particularly for the father, which a loving, happy sex life can help to diminish or even do away with altogether. A continued healthy sex life throughout the time of conception and early pregnancy can sometimes prevent any such problems occurring at all. Take the case of a husband who, however irrationally, finds himself becoming jealous of the new baby growing inside his wife. If a previously good sex life becomes less and less frequent and obviously less enjoyable to his wife, he may understandably resent this and put all the blame on the baby. He may feel shut out from his wife's love, and unnecessarily pushed aside. Particularly with a first baby, he may feel displaced as 'number one' in his partner's life and consequently feel rejected and unloved. This would be a sad case indeed, and quite unnecessary, because even if a woman cannot bring herself to participate in intercourse itself, there is usually some way around the situation. There are many ways of pleasing your partner which do not necessarily involve the sex act itself. During pregnancy is as good a time as any to experiment a bit, and a loving relationship need not be totally reliant on intercourse itself. There are many more tender, loving gestures that are equally nice. It is certainly important to voice your feelings at this time, and to consider any sexual problems you encounter as a joint difficulty, not something to be attributed to either partner alone. There can be no apportioning of 'blame' in such a situation, it is just something that each couple has to work out for themselves. Be honest with each other, talk things through, discuss the situation, and explain your own feelings. Then you will have a good base on which to build a lasting solution to the changes you encounter in your life-style and your sex life.

Sex can be good for the foetus too

There is some indication (not yet fully understood or proven beyond doubt) that sex can be good for the growing baby inside you. It is thought by some doctors that regular sexual involvement, especially during the early stages of pregnancy when the foetus itself is still forming, encourages a good blood supply to the uterus. During sexual intercourse, and especially if the woman has an orgasm, all the sexual organs become engorged with blood. This is thought to ensure an adequate supply of the nutrients and oxygen that are needed by the growing baby, and may help it to satisfactorily implant itself into the wall of the womb. Frequency of sex need not differ from whatever was normal for each couple before conception took place. If you are at all worried about making love during your pregnancy, you can avoid having sex during the times when your first three periods would have been due under normal circumstances, as statistically speaking these are the most likely times for miscarriage to occur.

The rising libido

Pregnancy can be the most intensely sexual time of your life or it can be the most sexually limited time, depending on how you feel both physically and mentally. Let's look on the bright side first. Some lucky people find that the state of pregnancy enhances their relationship with their partner to a wonderful degree. This is especially true when the baby has been planned in advance and loved from the start. Even with an unplanned pregnancy, once the idea of a new baby has sunk in it can bring the parents closer together and be a real blessing in this way. A love child such as this can draw its parents closer together and can heal up any cracks in the relationship that might have existed previously. Most men find the enlarging, pregnant shape of their wife very attractive and sexy. Pregnancy often produces a radiant, shining, healthy look in an expectant mother, which is very becoming and can transform a formerly dull complexion into a vivid, translucently clear skin and healthy appearance. Most men are attracted by the gently rounding figure of their woman as the pregnancy begins to show, and many couples find the idea of making love with the roundness of a longed-for child between them a truly erotic experience. Some men find that the more rounded and pregnant their wives become, the more sexually appealing they are. It is also thought that pregnancy produces certain 'pheromones' in women which are sexually arousing to men – your very own, sexy, enticing perfume.

Once you know for sure that you have conceived, any barriers between you which were caused by the interference of contraception will disappear. All contraceptives interfere with lovemaking to some degree. Barrier methods can be messy and off-putting for some, while the pill can give you headaches and can cause loss of libido. Traditional, natural, rhythm methods always involve an uneasy feeling that you could easily conceive by mistake, and this in itself can be nerve-racking and can make sex less enjoyable. Some women cannot enjoy sex much at all because they have this constant fear of becoming pregnant unwillingly and unexpectedly. If pregnancy does occur in such a case, then after the initial shock of getting used to the idea a woman may feel released from these responsibilities and start enjoying sex in full. Once the tenseness and strain caused by the necessity to use contraception is removed, lovemaking sometimes takes on a new excitement for both partners. Once a woman is pregnant there is nothing much else to be done, so she might as well enjoy herself and the pregnancy, unless she is seriously considering an abortion. All women experience a greater physical sensitivity during pregnancy. This can work either in your favour or against you in your sexual relationship. You may find that any physical contact at all turns you off, or alternatively you may become tuned in to the new frequency of touch and find yourself becoming very much more responsive to the extra sensitivity. Your breasts will become very much more sensitive to touch, and to any pressure from your partner. If you find this unpleasant during lovemaking, now may be the time to forgo the usual 'missionary' position and try something else that will not involve your partner lying directly on top of you. You may find this extra sensitivity of the breasts quite erotic, provided you are approached delicately and sympathetically.

There is one further good role that sex could play in your pregnancy should your baby become overdue. Most doctors are reluctant to allow any pregnancy to continue for more than two weeks after the expected date of delivery, and at this point many of them favour artificial induction of the baby, using intravenous chemicals to start off contractions. It is a shame to have to resort to this method when all it may take to start off labour is a gentle session of lovemaking with your partner. Many couples I know have used this method of helping to start overdue labour, with great success. Lovemaking is sometimes all it takes to start things naturally, and it's a much nicer way of helping your baby into the world than any other.

The diminishing libido

Although some women find they feel much more sexy during pregnancy, others feel just the opposite. Some women shy away from sex at this time for a variety of reasons, and if this is the case for you, don't worry. It is quite a common occurrence, and it need not put an undue strain on your relationship with your man provided you both take time to talk things through, and provided you make sure your partner understands the real reasons behind the change and does not just feel left out and rejected. It is up to you to continue being a loving, thoughtful partner by showing your affection in other ways, and by letting him know that you are not rejecting him because he is no longer attractive to you. The male ego can be a delicate thing and is easily dented, so take care to explain the real reasons behind your lack of interest in bed. Don't automatically assume that just because you didn't feel sexy during one pregnancy the same thing will happen in subsequent pregnancies. Each pregnancy is different, and each time your feelings will be different too.

One of the most common reasons for loss of libido in early pregnancy is simply that you may feel so awful. Most women suffer from morning sickness to some degree, and this does not necessarily strike just during the early mornings, but can also be a nuisance throughout the day and in the evenings too. On top of this you may be feeling particularly tired and lethargic. This is not your fault – it is due to the enormous changes that your body is going through, and does not mean that you are just being lazy. These two factors combined are enough to turn anybody off. If you explain this to your man carefully, it is up to him to be sympathetic and understanding. He should not force the issue, or make a big thing out of it. He should not moan or make a fuss. After all, you are in the process of creating a new life between you, and concessions will have to be made on both sides. The symptoms will probably disappear after the first twelve to fourteen weeks of pregnancy, and it is likely that you will return to your old self. Most women feel at their best during the middle months of pregnancy – they are still able to move about fairly easily, while the dreaded sickness should no longer be a problem.

A sensation of tenderness in the breasts and over your abdomen is another well-known symptom of pregnancy, and this can also cause a disinterest in sex. Sometimes your breasts can be so tender that any pressure on them or any physical approach from your husband is very irritating and off-putting. You may not be able to bear him touching you at all at this time. Alternatively, you may only object to the pressure caused by the weight of your man on top of you (this used to give me instant heartburn). In this case use your imagination and try a different position which does not involve your man lying directly on top of you. There are many variations; just experiment a little and you are bound to find something you both like. One of the simplest alternatives is to swop positions, so that you are sitting or lying on top of your man. This has the added advantage that you can control the depth of penetration by your husband, and as time goes by and your bump increases in size you can sit, rather than lie, on top of your partner. Don't forget about oral sex – now is the time to experiment if you haven't tried it before. You may find it the perfect answer to your problem.

If your baby was not planned but happened by mistake or error, you may well feel resentful at first. This is understandable, and it can also turn a woman away from sex. You may blame your pregnancy on your husband's recklessness, or his lack of care and control. Or you may even suspect that he wanted you to have another baby even though he knew you were against the idea. All these feelings need talking through with your husband before the block which is stopping you enjoying sexual relations can be lifted.

It is quite reasonable to suppose that a decreased libido during pregnancy is a natural phenomenon. After all, as already mentioned, most other mammals refuse sex at this time. In the evolution of animals and of man, sexual desire is a method of ensuring the survival of the species. Sexual desire is often heightened in the female during her most fertile time, and naturally decreases afterwards, either when she has become pregnant or when she is no longer in a fertile state. Once conception has taken place, which is what nature had intended, there is little logical reason from nature's point of view for sexual desire to continue.

Some women find that although they still have some sexual desire and are sexually receptive, the feeling is not as strong as it was previously and gradually diminishes further as the pregnancy progresses. For instance, a woman who usually experiences an orgasm every time intercourse takes place might still feel like making love but might not feel like reaching a climax. Some women avoid orgasm during pregnancy because they suspect it could damage the baby somehow, or possibly cause a miscarriage, but this is most unlikely. The baby is very well protected *in utero* and a healthy foetus is not easily dislodged. If you have a miscarriage soon after making love, don't blame yourself. You would probably have had a miscarriage anyway, whether or not you had made love at this time – spontaneous abortion is nature's way of sorting out the healthy from the unhealthy, and of making sure that only the strongest progeny survive.

During the last three months of pregnancy, intercourse becomes particularly difficult because of the sheer size of the baby inside you, and because you may feel lumpy, uncomfortable and unattractive at this time. At this stage you may suffer from heartburn, and from various other minor ailments which can combine to turn you off. However, if you still feel like making love, carry on. It cannot damage the baby, so enjoy yourself without feeling guilty. If you are too tired at night, try having sex in the morning, or in the afternoon, or whenever you feel like it. Pregnancy gives your sexual life a whole new rhythm, so just accept whatever happens. Your husband should try to go along with whatever you desire, and your aim should be not to neglect him unkindly.

Husbands can suffer from loss of libido too

The husband of a pregnant woman may himself sometimes suffer from a diminished libido. He may feel that his wife is very vulnerable at this time, and that any sexual interference may damage the baby or cause a miscarriage. This is very unlikely indeed, as already stated, but nevertheless it is a common, mistaken idea. Some husbands just don't want to disturb their baby in its cocoon within its mother. They may feel like intruders in this situation. Later on in pregnancy, when the baby is moving around a lot and is kicking frequently, your husband may feel the baby moving inside you during intercourse. He may not like this sensation. He may feel abhorrence at being able to feel the baby in this way, and it may make him squeamish. (Some husbands, however, may be delighted by it.) Some men may feel that the baby is kicking against *them*, in protest at being disturbed. Again this is most unlikely, but if your husband expresses some distaste, try to be understanding and helpful rather than mocking or laughing at him.

The contraindications

You should not indulge in sexual activities during pregnancy in any of the following circumstances:

1. If you have had a previous miscarriage, you should avoid sexual intercourse until after the fourteenth week of pregnancy.

2. If you have had several previous miscarriages, you should not have sexual intercourse unless and until your doctor decides that it is safe for you to do so. Your doctor's decision on this will depend on your individual case.

3. If you have a threatened miscarriage (i.e. bleeding, or severe abdominal pains) at any stage of pregnancy, sexual intercourse must stop. This can happen at any time during a pregnancy, but you must be especially diligent about it if it occurs during the last third of a pregnancy, because every day your baby remains inside you at this stage enhances its chance of being mature enough for survival if born.

10

Your Body after Birth

Although your whole life will revolve around your baby once it is born, you will soon want to turn some attention to regaining your figure and getting back into good physical shape. The womb itself is a wonderfully efficient organ – in most cases it completely contracts back to its former shape and size within eight weeks, the greater part of this taking place during the first two weeks after birth. Regaining your previous figure completely, and getting your stomach muscles elastic again, can take a little longer than this. After all, your body has been changing, growing and evolving for nine months in readiness for the birth of your baby, and you can't expect it just to snap back into shape again immediately. However, most of the bulges and sagging muscles should have very nearly disappeared by the time the baby is six months old. Depending on how much weight you put on during your pregnancy, you may or may not have some excess weight to lose afterwards. Don't be too despondent about this – it will take a little time for your body to revive itself again. On the day your baby is born you will automatically lose about a stone, and possibly a little more. This automatic weight loss is made up simply from the weight of the baby, the placenta, the waters that surrounded the baby inside the womb, and a quantity of blood which is lost during the delivery. This loss is immediate. During the next few weeks you will continue to lose a little more weight as your body returns to its former state. Your womb will continue to shrink back to its normal, non-pregnant size, and if you were prone to water retention as your pregnancy progressed you will now lose the excess water that was deposited in your tissues. After the first twelve weeks or so, you will be able to see whether you need to start counting the calories to lose a few more pounds, or whether you are already close enough to your previous weight not to have to bother to slim. If you find you are still a bit overweight, now is the time to get to grips with the situation and start to do something about it.

Breastfeeding can also make a difference. If you don't breastfeed, your breasts will gradually decrease in size and you will lose another couple of pounds as this happens. If you do breastfeed, you may well find this an advantage in regaining your previous weight for various reasons. Firstly, as the baby suckles at the breast certain hormones are released which speed up the process of the womb returning to its former size and shape. Secondly, when you are feeding the baby yourself you use up quite a few more calories per day, which are used in the production of milk for the baby. (If you are breastfeeding you may need up to 2,700 calories per day.) Don't forget that during pregnancy your body has already laid down some extra calories in the form of fat. This store of calories is used to make milk for the baby in the first few weeks after birth. So if you want to take the easiest route to losing that store of fat, breastfeeding can help you. If you breastfeed, your body will automatically use up the extra fat that was laid down for that purpose, and as the weeks go by you will lose a little more weight (provided you don't overeat at the same time). While you are breastfeeding it is important to keep eating a balanced diet, rich in the things your baby needs, but this diet need not be particularly high in calories. You will certainly need to keep eating plenty of protein, for example lean meat, poultry, fish, eggs and cheese, and you will also need lots of fresh vegetables and some fresh fruit. You will still need some carbohydrates, such as bread and cereals, but you can keep these to a minimum as your aim is to use up the fat already laid down in your body instead of eating even more of it (excess carbohydrate in the diet is turned into fat and deposited in the body). Most importantly, make sure you drink plenty when you are breastfeeding – you will need about four pints of liquid each day, preferably unadulterated, unsweetened drinks such as fruit juices, weak tea, herb teas, or just plain water.

Don't forget about your posture once the baby is born. Your posture will alter again after the birth because you will no longer have to allow for the lump on your front, which previously threw you off balance and tilted your pelvis forward. Now you are back to normal, but make an effort to keep your posture straight and erect. A bad posture makes flabby muscles look even more flabby, while a good posture goes a long way towards disguising a sagging figure and flabby muscles, especially around the waist.

The muscles

Unless you have had complications during your labour, there is no reason why you should not start to exercise your stretched muscles gently as soon as you feel like it, ideally on the day after the birth. There are two different sets of muscles which have been distended, strained and stretched by the processes of pregnancy and birth, and each set of muscles needs toning up again individually in order to get back to normal quickly.

The first set of muscles that needs to be concentrated on are the muscles of the pelvic floor. These will have been stretched a lot to allow your baby to be born, and they are important because they need a reasonable amount of tone in them before you will be fit to carry on with everyday lifting of any sort. (When you lift a fairly heavy weight, your pelvic floor muscles tense up to support your bladder, uterus, rectum, and other internal organs, and they need to be firm to stop everything sagging.) If you needed stitches in your perineum after the birth, you may find that the pelvic floor exercises are just a little bit uncomfortable to begin with. Don't use this as an excuse not to do them, but take care to do them gently, slowly and gradually, carefully building up a routine, as and when you feel you are ready. The exercises to re-tone your pelvic floor muscles are the same ones that were used to strengthen the pelvic floor during pregnancy, and can be found on pp. 175–6. (You can do all the pelvic floor exercises straight after the birth, with the exception of No. 5, 'Sexual activity'. Most doctors recommend abstention from any sexual activity for at least six weeks after the birth of a baby, until the pelvic floor and the pelvic organs have had time to heal properly. However, once the baby is six weeks old, sexual activity is a very good way to strengthen your pelvic floor muscles again. Gentle intercourse can start again after six weeks, as soon as you feel able and in the mood.)

The second set of muscles that need re-toning are the muscles of the abdomen. Obviously these have been stretching and expanding for several months, and they may well take several more months to regain all their elasticity. These tummy muscles will feel very flabby to begin with, especially during the first few days after the birth. Some women describe their stomach muscles during the first few days after delivery as 'jelly-like'. Don't worry, they will not stay like this for ever. Over the next few days and weeks the tummy muscles will firm up a little of their own accord, but if you really want to regain the sort of muscle tone you had before pregnancy you must exercise these muscles properly.

First week

During the first few days after the birth, the most important exercises to do are those for the pelvic floor. Some women find that they have trouble urinating after a birth, and can lose the sensation of knowing when they need to pass water for a day or so. If you conscientiously practise using your pelvic floor muscles, this should help you regain control more quickly and effectively. During the first week after the birth you can also try some gentle exercises to help get your stomach muscles flat and working properly again. To begin with these should be fairly limited and gentle, but just a little time spent on them every day will soon make your tummy muscles less saggy and encourage the return of some tone.

1. *Thinking thin*. Lie on your back with your legs together and your arms by your sides. Contract the muscles in your

tummy so that it flattens, hold for 5 seconds, then relax. Repeat 5 times. After a few days you will be able to progress to trying this exercise standing up or as you are walking along. Imagine you are walking along a beach wearing a swimming costume, in full view of lots of thin people who are all staring at you. Think yourself thin. Pull your tummy in as much as you can, try to make your waist as small as possible, really pull those muscles inwards so that your stomach is quite flat. Hold for 5 seconds, then relax. Repeat 5 times.

2. *Knee reaches*. Lie on your back with your legs together and knees bent, keeping your feet resting on the floor and resting your hands on the tops of your legs. Slowly raise your head a little, and try to reach for your knees with your hands. Reach a little further, lifting your shoulders up too. (You probably won't be able to reach your knees at this stage, but just aim for your knees and feel the pull on your tummy muscles, which should be contracting tightly.) Slowly return to your former position. Repeat 5 times.

Second week

Once your baby is one week old, and your tummy muscles have started to respond a little to the previous week's gentle movements and have got a little strength back in them, you will be able gradually to increase the number of times you repeat each exercise and to introduce a couple of new ones into your routine. Gradually increase the number of times you do exercises 1 and 2 above by one extra time each day until you have worked up to 30 times daily. As soon as you feel fit and able you may add the following exercises.

3. *Leg lifting*. Lie down on your back, legs together, arms by your side. Slowly lift one leg into the air, then slowly bring it down again. Do the same with the other leg. Repeat the whole exercise 5 times. When this gets too easy for you after a few more weeks, as you begin to get some strength back in your muscles, try lifting both legs together instead of singly.

4. *Sit ups*. Lie on your back, legs straight, arms by your sides.

Slowly raise your head and torso until you reach a sitting position. Then slowly return to your former position. Repeat 5 times.

5. *Side swings*. Stand up straight, feet slightly apart, about nine inches away from a wall and with your back to it. Keeping your feet firmly in the same position, swing your torso round and place your hands flat against the wall. Then swing round in the other direction, again placing your hands flat against the wall. Repeat 5 times.

Losing any left-over weight

As already mentioned, your body will change back to something not too different from its normal state only gradually, over a period of weeks after your baby is born. Of course your body will never return completely to its pre-pregnant state, but any remaining differences should be very minor, and not noticeable to anyone but yourself (and possibly your husband). Your tummy may not be *quite* so flat and taut as previously, your waist may not be quite so tiny, and perhaps your breasts may not be quite so firm as before, but these tiny physical differences really shouldn't be enough to be noticeable by any of your friends or by outsiders. If you find that your figure is still drastically different six months or so after the birth, you have probably retained some of your extra weight and will need to lose a few pounds to get back to normal again. It is worth making the effort to regain your former weight and figure at this stage, especially if you are planning to have another baby at some time in the future. If you wait until after a second or subsequent baby to lose the excess weight you put on with your first, it will be much more difficult to shift, and the problem may be compounded by each successive pregnancy. For example, if you have an excess half a stone to lose after your first pregnancy, you will probably not find it too difficult to shed if you tackle it fairly soon. Most people find they can lose half a stone quite easily. But suppose you wait until after another pregnancy, when you may put on *another* half a stone too much and end up with a whole stone to lose as a result? You will find it much more difficult to lose this larger amount all in one go, as you will be likely to lose interest half-way and be tempted to give up before you reach your goal. By the time your baby is six months old you should be able to fit back into your old jeans and waisted skirts comfortably. If not, check your actual weight against the desirable weight given on p. 13.

It is a good idea to allow at least six months for your figure to adjust after the birth – it may easily take that long to regain your former shape and size. If you are breastfeeding, you should not try to restrict your calorie intake before this anyway, as for the first four months your baby will be relying solely on your body for all its nourishment. By the time the baby is six months old, however, it should be gradually adding various solid foods to its diet and will no longer be relying totally on you for its meals. At this stage you can restrict your own diet without fear of affecting your baby's food supply. (In fact, amply nutritious breast milk is usually miraculously formed from the mother's body regardless of her own diet, but this means that you may suffer the effects of bad nutrition if you breastfeed and diet at the same time, because the baby may use your own stores of nutrients if you are not eating enough to satisfy both your baby's needs and your own. This can lead to you becoming unnecessarily run down and overtired, and you need all the energy and zip you can muster to look after and feed an infant.)

The only sure way to guarantee weight loss is to restrict your daily calorie intake. The best number of calories to allow yourself is usually 1,000 per day – this is generally thought to be both enough to ensure adequate nutrition and few enough to sustain a steady weight loss without making you feel too hungry. How you take those calories each day is entirely up to you, but nowadays the emphasis in slimming is on a high fibre diet. This helps you to feel fuller for longer, thereby beating the recurring hunger pangs associated with other diets. If you follow the general rules for good nutrition in Chapter 2 and the advice about diet in Chapter 4 ('pre-conception diet', which in fact is also a good post-natal diet and indeed an excellent healthy diet to follow for the rest of your life), you will be following a naturally high fibre diet anyway and so will automatically gain the benefits of high fibre eating. As long as you stick to 1,000 calories per day you will lose weight steadily and surely. Some people prefer to allow themselves more calories than this, up to 1,500 calories per day. You will still lose weight with this daily calorie level, but it will be at a much slower pace; while you will not feel so hungry and may find it easier to stick to your diet, your slower weight loss may make you lose enthusiasm and interest and it will take you much longer to reach your target weight. Whatever calorie level you choose, my advice is to try to avoid processed, adulterated foods and to eat only natural, fresh foods whenever possible.

Slimmer's support plan

If you have any trouble staying within your chosen calorie allowance for several weeks (and let's face it, most of us do at some stage during a diet), here are a few tried and tested tips to help you persevere and overcome any moments of weakness.

1. Keep a bowl of ready prepared salad vegetables in the fridge, to munch when you are feeling hungry between meals. Chopped raw carrot, celery, mushrooms, tomatoes and cucumber are all good, and all are very low in calories so you can eat as much as you like without bothering to count up the calorie total.

2. Have a hot, low-calorie drink when you are feeling weak-willed and fancy something more substantial but forbidden. Hot drinks always *seem* to be more satisfying and filling than cold ones. Try black tea or coffee, or indulge in a range of delicious herbal teas. You can buy them in one-portion, individual tea-bag sachets for convenience, and they have no calories whatsoever. A teaspoon of savoury yeast extract dissolved in water is also very good, and the hearty, savoury flavour can ward off a craving for something sweet. It's nutritious too!

3. Use skimmed milk in place of whole milk throughout your diet. You won't notice the difference in taste, but you will save quite a lot of calories.

4. Use fruit as a treat. Allow yourself a specially sweet fruit, such as a peach or some fresh pineapple, as a between-meals treat. Or make yourself a fresh fruit salad and add a few pieces of dried fruit to make it extra sweet – dried dates are particularly sweet, and one or two go a long way in a fruit salad.

5. Don't forget about yogurt – it can make a delicious low-calorie snack. But make sure you buy only unsweetened yogurt, or make your own (it's cheaper).

6. Eat foods that are high in natural fibre, as these help to fill you up more and will keep you feeling full for longer. Use only wholewheat flour and bread, and try brown rice instead of white.

7. Eat your largest meal of the day at breakfast time, and your smallest meal for supper. If you eat most of your calories during the first half of the day, this will give you more opportunity of burning them off again as you go about your daily work or routine. A large breakfast will also provide you with adequate energy to enable you to cope at your busiest time of day. If you eat your largest meal in the evening and then sit down to read or to watch television, you will have little opportunity of burning up many of the calories.

8. Keep a weekly progress chart of your weight loss on a prominent wall, where other people can easily see it. This will encourage you to persevere with your diet so that your wall chart will look successful, and it will be obvious to everyone who sees it that you are really winning your battle against excess weight. Then you will be less likely to lapse into lethargy and high calorie sloth.

9. Carry a photograph of yourself at your very fattest at all times. When you feel tempted by biscuits or fattening cakes or buns, look at your photo and you will find extra determination to stick to your diet.

10. Stick a picture of a slim, lithe model in a bikini inside

the door of the cupboard where you keep those foods that are the most difficult to resist, as a warning to resist temptation.

11. Slim with a friend. Most people find it easier to keep to a diet if they have another person to slim with, as this gives mutual encouragement. If you have a friend or neighbour who also wants to lose weight, why not join forces and slim together? Then you can compare weight loss and exchange favourite slimming recipes. Also it is good to have a friend whom you can ring up in moments of weakness to remind you of your goal and to fire your enthusiasm once again when your resistance is low.

12. If you have a lot of weight to lose, allow yourself a special treat for every half a stone you lose. A new dress, a hairdo, or a trip to the cinema or theatre perhaps (but *not* a celebration meal out!). This will give you something to look forward to, and give extra determination to stay on your diet in order to lose the next half stone.

13. Take up a new hobby. Don't lounge around the kitchen feeling sorry for yourself – boredom is one of the likeliest diet breakers of all. Take an interest in something different, for example knitting, sewing, embroidery, photography, learning French, swimming, collecting stamps, or whatever takes your fancy. Whenever you feel as if you may break your diet, move away from the kitchen and absorb yourself in your new hobby.

14. Make sure you get out of the house at least once every day. It is easy to over-eat if you've nothing better to do. Make sure you have a change of scenery now and then. Get out and about. Go for a walk in the country or in the nearest local park. A new baby needn't hinder you in this, as babies need fresh air too.

Addresses

The following pages list addresses of some organizations which give useful information and provide leaflets and other services which are relevant and helpful to the pregnant woman.

The Maternity Alliance, 309 Kentish Town Road, London NW5 2TJ (Tel. 01 267 3255). The Maternity Alliance is a voluntary organization campaigning for the rights of mothers, fathers and babies. Their aims include improving the health care given to families before conception, during pregnancy and childbirth, and in the following twelve months. They want to improve the social support given to pregnant women and new parents, and financial support for poorer pregnant women and parents. They also aim to improve the legal rights of parents during and after pregnancy. They have a good range of leaflets and pamphlets on all these aspects.

Foresight, The Association for the Promotion of Preconceptual Care, c/o Mrs Peter Barnes, The Old Vicarage, Church Lane, Witley, Godalming, Surrey GU8 5PN (Tel Wormley (042879) 4500 between 9.30 a.m. and 7.30 p.m.). Foresight has been formed to see that all possible steps are taken to ensure that every baby enters the world free from congenital deformity and mental damage and in perfect health. The concept embraces two plans of action; firstly to take steps to secure optimal health and nutritional status in both prospective parents, prior to conception, and secondly to instigate research aimed at the identification and removal of potential health hazards to foetal development in the external environment in which the mother will carry the child. To make this concept a reality, Foresight are in the process of setting up a nationwide network of clinics where couples can go to discuss preconceptual care and diet. Please enclose SAE for details.

The National Childbirth Trust, 9 Queensborough Terrace, London W2 3TB (Tel. 01 221 3833). The National Childbirth Trust are concerned with education and preparation for parenthood. They have a comprehensive list of literature, available on request, on all aspects of pregnancy and childbirth.

The Society to Support Home Confinements, Margaret Whyte, 17 Laburnum Avenue, Durham City (Tel. Durham 61325). This society has all the advice and details necessary to help you if you require a home delivery for your baby. Please enclose a large SAE.

Maternity Defence Fund, 33 Castle Close, Henley-in-Arden, Warwickshire. The purpose of the fund is to raise cash to support test cases of alleged misconduct against patients by professionals working in maternity units, so that parents' rights can be established in law. They are willing to advise parents of the kind of action they can take following their experiences in pregnancy, childbirth and postnatally. They aim to assist parents to obtain early legal opinion.

The Association for Improvements in the Maternity Services, Mrs Christine Rodgers, 163 Liverpool Road, London N1 0RF. AIMS exists as a pressure group covering all aspects of the maternity services. It is made up mostly of mothers, together with a few professionals who are interested in the consumer's views. Their aims are to bring about improvements in the maternity services by informing parents of the choices available, and by informing the DHSS and the medical profession of parents' views. They have many regional and local groups, and publish a quarterly newsletter crammed with reports, reviews and news of any changes in obstetric policy.

The Birth Centre, PO Box 115, London SW11 6BQ (Tel. 01 223 4747). The Birth Centre gives support to those people in London who seek an alternative to the ever-increasing mechanization of birth. They also have many regional centres which provide the same services in other areas. They have a good information service on all aspects of hospital and home birth, and publish a quarterly newsletter about birth and related topics. They are actively encouraging others to set up more regional centres throughout the country.

The Association of Radical Midwives, The Secretary, Lakefield, 8a The Drive, Wimbledon SW 19. ARM is, its members stress, first and foremost a support and study group, not a pressure group. Their work is mainly among their fellow midwives and other professionals in the field of maternity care, to promote a more sensitive and informed attitude towards the women and babies they care for. They also have regional groups, which are autonomous and free to arrange meetings, speakers, films, etc. according to local need. They publish a quarterly newsletter which is packed full of interestingly written and informative articles and discussions. Mainly aimed at the medical profession, but others are welcome to join too.

The Health Education Council, 78 New Oxford Street, London WC1A 1AH (Tel. 01 637 1881). The HEC have a wealth of information concerning general health care and fitness.

Family Doctor Publications, BMA House, Tavistock Square, London WC1H 9JP (Tel. 01 387 9721). This organization has a very comprehensive list of pamphlets concerning many different aspects of health care, including several about pregnancy and childbirth, childcare and management, sex education and psychology. They are all available by mail order from the above address. Write to them for a list of titles and details of prices.

ASH, 5–11 Mortimer Street, London W1N 7RH (Tel. 01 637 9843). ASH (Action on Smoking and Health) have publications helpful to those who want to give up smoking, which is advisable if you want to become, or already are, pregnant. Send SAE for details.

The Family Planning Information Service, 27/35 Mortimer Street, London W1N 7RJ (Tel. 01 636 7866). The FPIS are able to supply advice and information on methods of contraception. They provide a phone-in advice service on the above telephone number, and answer letters on contraception and sexual and personal relationships. They also produce leaflets and other publications on birth control and related topics. One leaflet, 'When you have had your baby', is aimed particularly at new mothers and their contraceptive needs. The pill leaflet contains a section about using a barrier method before trying to conceive.

The Association for Spina Bifida and Hydrocephalus, Tavistock House North, Tavistock Square, London WC1 9HJ (Tel. 01 388 1382). ASBAH was formed in 1966 to assist all those born with spina bifida and/or hydrocephalus and their families. There are now more than 90 local branches in England, Wales and Northern Ireland. Support is channelled through social work support and welfare grants, advisory services on education, training, employment aids and equipment, accommodation and leisure. ASBAH runs social development and independence training courses, and also have a young people's group called LIFT. The association also actively supports research into the causes of spina bifida and hydrocephalus.

Calorie Chart

Food	Calories per oz/ fl oz/28 g	Food	Calories per oz/ fl oz/28g
Almonds, shelled	170	Bran	56
Anchovy fillets	45	Brazil nuts	177
Apple, eating or cooking	10	Bread, wholewheat	66
dried rings	70	white	62
juice	13	Broccoli	5
Apricot, fresh	6	Brussels sprouts	5
dried	50	Buckwheat	95
Arrowroot powder	100	Bulghur, cracked wheat	102
Artichokes, globe	4	Butter	210
Jerusalem	5	Buttermilk	10
Asparagus	5		
Aubergine	5	Cabbage	4
Avocado pear, flesh only	62	Carob flour	100
		Carrots	5
Bacon, grilled	130	Cashew nuts	161
Banana, flesh only	22	Cauliflower	3
dried	75	Celeriac	4
Barley, raw	100	Celery	2
cooked	33	Cheese, Stilton	130
Beans, baked tinned	20	Brie	88
broad, boiled	14	Camembert	88
butter, boiled	26	Cheddar	120
French, boiled	2	cottage	28
haricot, boiled	26	cream	125
lentils, boiled	27	curd	40
mung, boiled	29	Edam	88
mung, fresh beansprouts	10	Gouda	100
red kidney, boiled	32	Parmesan	118
runner, boiled	5	Cherries	11
soya, boiled	37	Chestnuts, shelled	48
Beef, lean meat	55	Chicken, lean meat	42
minced	63	meat and skin	62
Beetroot, cooked	12	Chickpeas, cooked	41
Blackberries	8	Chicory	3
Blackcurrants	8	Chinese leaves	3

Calorie Chart

Food	Calories per oz/floz/28g	Food	Calories per oz/floz/28g
Cocoa powder	90	Halibut	28
Coconut, fresh	100	Ham, lean meat	60
desiccated	170	Hazel nuts	110
milk	6	Heart	28
Cod	25	Herring	52
Coffee, per cup, black	0	Honey	81
Coley	23	Jam, average	78
Cornflour	100		
Corn oil	254	Kidney, raw	27
Corn on the cob, kernels only	35	Kippers	33
Courgettes	4	Lamb, lean meat	55
Crab, meat only	35	Leeks	8
Cream, double	127	Lemon	4
single	60	juice	2
Cucumber	3	Lentils	27
Currants	70	Lettuce	3
		Lime	8
Damsons	10	Liver	55
Dates, fresh	30	Lobster	33
dried	70	Lychees	18
Duck, meat only	53	Macaroni, boiled	32
meat and skin	90	Mackerel	52
Eel	55	Malt extract	100
Eggs, size 1	95	Mango	18
size 3	80	Marrow	2
size 5	70	Mayonnaise	206
yolk, size 1	75	Melon	4
white, size 1	20	Milk, whole	18
Endive	3	skimmed, liquid	9
		skimmed, dried	100
Fennel	7	goats	20
Figs, dried	60	Molasses	72
Flour, wholewheat	90	Mushrooms	4
white	96	Mussels	25
Garlic	39	Nectarines	14
Gherkins	5	Noodles, cooked	33
Goose	90		
Gooseberries	7	Oats	113
Grapes	17	Oil	255
juice	20	Okra	7
Grapefruit	6	Olives	25
Greengages	12	Onions	6
		Oranges	10
Haddock	25	juice	9

Pregnancy and Diet

Food	Calories per oz/floz/28g	Food	Calories per oz/floz/28g
Oysters	14	Salsify	5
		Sardines	50
Parsnips	15	Sauerkraut	5
Passionfruit	10	Semolina, raw	96
Pastry, shortcrust	130	Sesame seeds	160
Peaches	9	Soya sauce	20
Peanuts	160	Spinach	9
Peanut butter	176	Spring greens	3
Pears	10	Spring onions	10
Peas	15	Strawberries	7
Peppers, green or red	4	Sugar	112
Pheasant, lean meat	60	Sultanas	71
Pilchards	36	Sunflower seeds	168
Pineapple	13	Swede	5
juice	16	Sweet potato	24
Pistachio nuts	180		
Plaice	25	Tangerines	10
Plums	10	Tea, black, per cup	0
Pomegranate	19	Tomatoes	4
Popcorn, popped	108	juice	5
Pork, lean meat	65	Tripe	27
crackling	192	Trout	25
Potatoes	25	Tuna, in oil	60
Prawns	12	Turkey, lean meat	40
Prunes, dried	40	meat and skin	50
Pumpkin	4	Turnips	4
seeds	159		
		Veal	55
Quince	7	Venison	56
		Vinegar	1
Rabbit, lean meat	37		
Radishes	4	Walnuts	150
Raisins	70	Water chestnuts	23
Raspberries	7	Watercress	4
Redcurrants	6	Watermelon	4
Rhubarb	2	Wheatgerm	100
Rice, brown, boiled	35	Wheat, whole grains	95
Rye, flour	94		
		Yeast, dried	48
Salmon	50	fresh	15
		Yogurt	16

Index

Index

Index

PENGUIN COOKERY BOOKS

☐ *Mediterranean Cookbook* **Arabella Boxer**   £2.50

A gastronomic grand tour of the region: 'The best book on Mediterranean cookery I have read since Elizabeth David' – *Sunday Express*

☐ *Josceline Dimbleby's Book of Puddings, Desserts and Savouries*   £1.75

By the *Sunday Telegraph*'s popular cookery columnist, a book 'full of the most delicious and novel ideas for every type of pudding, from the tasty, filling family variety to exotic pastry concoctions' – *Lady*

☐ *Penguin Cordon Bleu Cookery*   £2.50

Find the highest quality of European cooking with a French accent in this classic Penguin cookery book, prepared by Rosemary Hume and Muriel Downes, co-principals of the English Cordon Bleu School.

☐ *A Concise Encyclopedia of Gastronomy* **André Simon**   £6.95

Expertly edited, with wit and wisdom, this is the most comprehensive survey ever published, and a treasure-house of good food.

☐ *Barbecues* **James F. Marks**   £1.95

From choosing your barbecue to smoke-cooking, and from tandoori chicken to pizza and bananas Diana – the new, updated edition of this bestselling handbook is indispensable to everyone wanting to dine out deliciously in their own back garden.

☐ *The Chocolate Book* **Helge Rubinstein**   £2.95

Part cookery book, part social history, this sumptuous book offers an unbeatable selection of recipes – chocolate cakes, ice-creams, pies, truffles, drinks and savoury dishes galore.

PENGUINS ON HEALTH, SPORT AND PHYSICAL FITNESS

☐ *The F-Plan* **Audrey Eyton**   £1.95

The book that started the diet revolution of the decade, *The F-Plan* is, quite simply, a phenomenon! Here Britain's top diet expert, Audrey Eyton, provides the recipes, menus and remarkable health revelations – everything you need to know to make that slim, fit future realistically possible.

☐ *The F-Plan Calorie Counter and Fibre Chart*
Audrey Eyton   £1.95

An indispensable companion to the F-Plan diet. High-fibre fresh, canned and packaged foods are listed, there's a separate chart for drinks, *plus* a wonderful new selection of effortless F-Plan meals.

☐ *The Arthritis Book*
Ephraim P. Engleman and Milton Silverman   £1.95

Written for patients and their families, this is a clear, expert and up-to-date handbook on arthritis, containing information on the latest drugs and treatments, and advice on how to cope.

☐ *Vogue Natural Health and Beauty*
Bronwen Meredith   £6.95

Health foods, yoga, spas, recipes, natural remedies and beauty preparations are all included in this superb, fully illustrated guide and companion to the bestselling *Vogue Body and Beauty Book*.

☐ *Alternative Medicine* **Andrew Stanway**   £3.25

From Acupuncture and Alexander Technique to Macrobiotics, Radionics and Yoga, Dr Stanway provides an expert and objective guide to thirty-two therapies, for everyone interested in alternatives to conventional medicine.

☐ *The Runner's Handbook*
Bob Glover and Jack Shepherd   £2.95

Supplementary exercises, injuries, women on the run, running shoes and clothing, training for competitions and lots more information is included in this internationally famous manual.

PENGUINS ON HEALTH, SPORT AND KEEPING FIT

☐ *Our Bodies Ourselves*
British edition by
Angela Phillips and Jill Rakusen £4.95

Described by the *Guardian* as 'The Bible of the women's health movement', this is the most successful book about women's health ever published, and it has already sold over one million copies worldwide.

☐ *Physical Fitness* £1.00

Containing the 5BX 11-minute-a-day plan for men, and the XBX 12-minute-a-day plan for women, this book illustrates the famous programmes originally developed by the Royal Canadian Air Force and now used successfully all over the world.

☐ *Vogue Guide to Skin Care, Hair Care and Make-up*
Felicity Clark £4.95

All three *Vogue* guides in a one-volume paperback! Here is professional advice from *Vogue* on all aspects of beauty care, to help you make the most of yourself and your looks.

☐ *The BTM Programme* **Don McLaren** £1.50

Devised by a medical expert and based on sound scientific principles, the Body Tone Maintenance Programme is a new, comprehensive plan of diet, exercise and relaxation that can be carried out with ease in your own home.

☐ *My Child Won't Sleep*
Jo Douglas and Naomi Richman £1.75

Persistent night waking, nightmares and fear of the dark are common problems with children, and *can* be overcome. This book, written by two authorities on childcare, provides practical advice and some well-tested methods for you to try.

☐ *Coping with Young Children*
Jo Douglas and Naomi Richman £1.75

A companion to *My Child Won't Sleep*, this is a helpful and essential guide to coping with the everyday problems which face most parents of young children.

PENGUINS ON HEALTH, SPORT AND KEEPING FIT

☐ *The Penguin Bicycle Handbook* **Rob van der Plas**   £3.95

Choosing a bicycle, maintenance, accessories, basic tools, safety, keeping fit – all these subjects and more are covered in this acclaimed, fully illustrated guide to the total bicycle lifestyle.

☐ *The Walker's Handbook* **Hugh Westacott**   £2.50

Maps, tents, clothes, boots, hostels, rights of way, National Parks, farmers, safety and first aid are all covered in this indispensable manual, plus new chapters on challenge walks and walking abroad.

☐ *Baby & Child* **Penelope Leach**   £7.95

A fully illustrated, expert and comprehensive handbook on the first five years of life. 'It stands head and shoulders above anything else available at the moment' – Mary Kenny in the *Spectator*

These books should be available at all good bookshops or news-agents, but if you live in the UK or the Republic of Ireland and have difficulty in getting to a bookshop, they can be ordered by post. Please indicate the titles required and fill in the form below.

NAME _____ BLOCK CAPITALS

ADDRESS _____

_____

_____

Enclose a cheque or postal order payable to The Penguin Bookshop to cover the total price of books ordered, plus 50p for postage. Readers in the Republic of Ireland should send £IR equivalent to the sterling prices, plus 67p for postage. Send to: The Penguin Book-shop, FREEPOST, Richmond-upon-Thames, Surrey TW9 1BR.

You can also order by phoning (01) 940 1802, and quoting your Barclaycard or Access number.

Every effort is made to ensure the accuracy of the price and availability of books at the time of going to press, but it is sometimes necessary to increase prices and in these circumstances retail prices may be shown on the covers of books which may differ from the prices shown in this list or elsewhere. This list is not an offer to supply any book.

This order service is only available to residents in the UK and the Republic of Ireland.